THE

MALE NURSE

SURVIVAL GUIDE

THE
MALE NURSE
SURVIVAL GUIDE

CHRIS LENGLE

DANCONIA GOLD

Disclaimer

This book is not meant as a substitute for professional or medical advice. The stories and lessons here are meant to be entertaining and insightful, but I am not responsible for your actions, decisions or feelings from reading this book.

Table of Contents

Dedicated to my parents who inspired me, my boys on the front lines, the nurses who always took care of me, and mostly my wife.

Jessica, this book (and I) wouldn't be worth a damn without you!

Introduction

It was just a normal change of shift like any other. The day shift and night shift nurses were at the station waiting to get started when one of them began telling a story about the new male nurse. She was describing for the other women a stupid comment he rattled off during their shift together yesterday. I do not remember the exact exchange, but I do remember how it fired up all the other female nurses. I was standing next to my buddy and fellow male nurse when I chuckled and said, "We had better teach this new guy how to survive around here, or he is going to get eaten alive!" We then began to joke about the women being lionesses and eating him like a little baby gazelle. Not long after that interaction, I trained a few nursing students for their clinical rotations. They followed me while we worked on the unit. I began to realize that nurses needed more than they are taught in nursing school. They needed a real, no-bull-shit survival guide!

This is the raw, real, and uncensored guide to surviving as a male nurse. Being a male in the female-dominated profession of nursing is dangerous. As you read each chapter of this book, you will learn the skills to not only survive but thrive. Whether you are thinking of becoming a nurse, a brand new nurse, or a seasoned professional, this book will give you entertaining and truthful insights on how to be a successful "murse."

At the time this book was written, there were over 4.2 million nurses in the United States. According to the National Nursing Workforce Survey, as of 2020, 9.4 percent of registered nurses in the United States are men.[1] That means for every one hundred nurses, ninety are women. You are in their world now!

I have filled this book with practical knowledge and skills learned through my fifteen-year nursing career. With my guidance, you are going to learn how to get the best schedules, get the best assignments, manage your time, survive crazy patients, and more. You will see the biggest pitfalls in nursing — and learn how to navigate them. You are going to learn the most important skills you need for a long, successful career as a male nurse.

This book is meant to be humorous; the goal is to have fun while you learn. This book is also meant to be relevant to nurses of all specialties so you can learn how to sustain a long nursing career. Nursing is a rewarding and exciting profession. It is full of opportunity and wonderful experiences. It is also hard! It will beat you up and spit you out. This book is designed to keep you in the game for a long time. While it is geared toward male nurses, any nurse will gain value from the wisdom found here. This book it is chock-full of practical advice, real-world experience, and time-tested frontline wisdom.

The Road Less Traveled

Believe it or not, I never thought I would be a male nurse. Only women are nurses, right? I especially didn't see myself writing a book about nursing. As I was working and orienting new nurses, I realized there are a lot of skills that we aren't taught when we enter this profession. The books and nursing schools teach you the rules, mechanics, pharmacology, etc. I wanted

---

1 Richard A. Smiley et al., "The 2020 National Nursing Workforce Survey," *Journal of Nursing Regulation* 12, no. 1, Supplement (April 1, 2021): S1-S96.

a book that told it like it was and gave real-life survival techniques that you won't learn in school. This is that book!

My journey started at seventeen years old, when I was wrestling with the rite of passage question, "What do I want to do for the rest of my life?" I enjoyed golfing, snowboarding, and hanging out with my friends. I had no idea what I wanted to do for a living. I wasn't even thinking about nursing.

It was 2004, and everyone in my small school was going to college for exciting professions. My parents asked me, "What do you want to do?" And I told them, "I don't know; I just want to make money and have free time." I was a good student and figured I could do anything.

I have to thank my parents for talking me into nursing. It was not a life calling. My mom had been a nurse for twenty some years at this point, and my dad was a big believer in me going to nursing school. They sat me down and pitched me the idea: "You can go to nursing school for two years, and the hospital will pay for it. You can come out with no debt, work three days a week, and make great money. You will always have a job and be far ahead of your friends going to college."

I heard "money and free time" . . . "OK, I'm in!"

Now, men in nursing are the minority now, but back then it was even weirder. The movie *Meet the Parents* debuted in 2000 and was a popular movie. I loved it! Ben Stiller's character was a male nurse. They poke fun at male nurses throughout the movie. His name was Gaylord Focker. So, of course, going into nursing it was . . . "Hey, Focker!"

I was the only guy going to nursing school in my graduating class. When I got there, I found out I was the youngest in the accelerated nursing program. I was eighteen years old, and the average age was thirty-five. They called me "Doogie" for *Doogie Howser, M.D.* I looked like I was twelve years old. There were about five other guys in the class of just over one hundred students. We naturally bonded together as men, and by graduation time, there were only around fifty students graduating . . . and only three guys left. I have a chapter on nursing school survival later in the book.

I will never forget being eighteen years old and having my first clinical experience at the nursing home. I was never a nursing assistant or spent any time in hospitals. I was now face to face with an eighty-year-old lady laying naked with all her goodies melting into the bed. She was just looking at me, and I was looking at her. I was hoping my face didn't show how I felt. It was my job to do the bed bath, and I was mortified. I have a twin brother who did not go to nursing school. I was thinking about how he was out having fun with our friends while I was scrubbing old ladies. "What the hell am I doing here?" I asked myself. Good news, I survived!

I graduated in 2006 at twenty years old. I had a whole new outlook on being a male nurse. Hell yes, I am a nurse; that was hard, and I made it! I was proud of it. It turned out that being Gaylord Focker had its perks.

I was saving lives and giving narcotics before I could even go out to the bar for a drink. Some of the elderly ladies would ask me if I was going to be a doctor. I didn't take offense because I am a guy and that is how they grew up: "Too much time and schooling for me, ma'am." Others would give a surprised look when a guy who looked like he was twelve years old came to take care of them. I would look surprised too, knowing how young I looked at the time.

Now, over fifteen years later, I am one of those old crotchety nurses like the ones I learned the ropes from. Being able to grow facial hair helped too. I have worked many units in many hospitals. I have worked all over the country, from sea to shining sea. I can diagnose *C. diff* from the smell at the door and eat my lunch right after that code brown without skipping a beat. I've had amazing mentors — and some terrible managers. I worked with the most caring and amazing nurses you can imagine. Some nurses, I still wonder how they passed nursing school. I am excited to share this knowledge with you.

I wish I had a book like this when I started. I wish I had someone to teach me the inner workings of being a nurse. I've kept every tip, secret, and insight short and actionable so you can put this book to use right away. My hope is that you return to it as a resource when you face different challenges throughout your career.

Welcome to the raw and real look at male nursing. Are you ready? Survival training starts now!

My Nursing Resume

Charge nurse and supervisor roles:

- Medical-surgical
- Stepdown-ICU
- ICU
- Telemetry
- Behavioral Health
- Orthopedics

Other Nursing:

- Camp nurse at a ski and snowboard camp in Oregon
- Local agency nurse floating between hospitals in Salt Lake City, Utah
- Computer medical data entry for Medicare compliance working from home
- Medical sales rep

Travel nursing; multiple assignments across the United States:

- San Diego, California: Prisoner floor, 2009
- Fresno, California: Bariatric surgical floor, 2016
- Bakersfield, California: Safety net hospital, 2019
- Hackensack, New Jersey: Critical staffing for coronavirus pandemic at long-term acute care facility, 2020
- Salt Lake City, Utah: Critical staffing for coronavirus pandemic, 2020–2021
- Onley, Maryland: Intermediate care unit, 2021–2022

Chapter 1

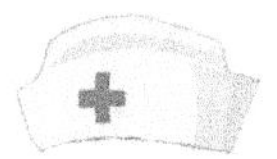

Welcome to the Jungle!

YOU'RE NOT IN THE HOSPITAL; YOU'RE IN THE JUNGLE NOW! Here, the women are the lionesses — and they rule this jungle. The outside world may have taught you differently, but this is their domain. If you only read this chapter, it was worth the price of this book.

There is a hierarchy in nursing, and it's best to learn it before it kills you. The lionesses will take amazing care of you if you know how to live in their pride. If you don't, then they will eat your face off! You must learn to walk among the lionesses, talk to them, and work with them. You must also know when not to talk or make any sudden moves to avoid their claws.

I experienced firsthand the lionesses taking down the mightiest of prey: alpha male wannabes who thought they could dominate the lionesses. These men might treat them poorly or open their mouths and say the wrong things. I have witnessed a new nurse manager only last a few weeks because he believed he was the new king of the jungle. The lionesses ate him up and spit him out. The alpha male may be the king in other domains, but this is the lionesses' jungle. You have to learn to live by their rules.

Working in a female-dominated area is both a skill and an art form. They will take great care of you and back you up if you respect them and abide by the rules. By the end of this book, you will be a master of the jungle. This is the way to do it.

The first thing you will learn quickly is that women love to talk about their family, life, and passions. They will tell you anything and everything going on in their lives at work. This is just their nature. This is especially true during night shifts. It was funny being a young man and a new nurse because I got the initial impression that all women just hated their husbands. I didn't have a lot of experience in this area, but they complained about them a lot. Their husbands didn't seem to do much right. I soon learned that most of the time this was just venting. They need to vent; it's their therapy. Most of them loved their husbands, even if they were dumbasses. We are all nurses in the trenches, so we trust each other to share.

The first rule to know is do not "guy advice" them or "mansplain" when they are venting. Women absolutely hate mansplaining! Guys like to give advice and try to fix problems. Women like to vent and talk out their problems. Trust me, it can be a difficult skill to master, as we love fixing things. Learn to be a good listener. Let the lionesses vent, and ask them questions. They will love you for it! Don't ever make them feel bad or guilty. I would suggest most of the time don't offer any advice at all. There is nothing women hate more than unsolicited advice. This is especially dangerous if they aren't even talking to you. I have watched male nurses butt in on lionesses' conversations. If looks could kill, they would be fresh meat.

These conversations go on at the nursing station, where many times you are just present and in listening range. The powerful skill to master is acting like you didn't hear a thing, even though you heard everything. Just keep on minding your business. Keep plugging along with your work. If you are prompted by them for your attention, just smile, laugh, and give some input. There were times when the female nurses would be talking about something raunchy and call over to say, "Wow, he is really getting an education over there." I would simply laugh and say, "Ohh, I'm just over here soaking up the knowledge." Laugh it off and be easy to have around, and they will love you for it. Don't be weird.

If you didn't already know, women have dirty minds. You will learn this quickly as a nurse. You will hear things that can make the raunchiest man blush. This is their jungle, and they feel like they can be open, have fun, and speak their mind. Listen and learn, but don't act judgmental, put off, or weird. If you are a sensitive man, then you best find a new line of work. Women have dirty minds and will break you. Just laugh these things off and keep on rolling. You may learn a thing or two.

Do not be a know-it-all is an important second rule. Sometimes women don't want to hear the answer, even if you know the answer. Offer up answers, but never make someone feel stupid. A good tactic I use often is presenting the answer in a question form. You want to act like you aren't 100 percent sure, even though you are. *"I'm pretty sure you can give that drug now?"* "I would *maybe* call the doctor for that?" "I *might* check their blood sugar again." It makes them feel like they are still in charge, and you aren't giving them orders. It sounds passive because it is passive . . . but it works.

The third rule is a big one: *do not gossip!* Like I said, a great skill to have is to hear everything, but do not participate. They have to know they can trust you. If you spread the dirty laundry around, then you will eventually be eaten. Become the trustworthy guy. Women will talk about each other, and there will be women who do not get along. Never pick a side, don't criticize one in front of the other, and be a neutral party. It can be difficult at times because women will attempt to win you over to their side. Do not give in. Jungle survival depends on them knowing you aren't a gossip.

The fourth rule is to not give away your secrets right away. Some men come onto a new unit and get all excited to share their life stories with everyone. You don't have to divulge your whole life story when you first arrive in the jungle. It makes you come off weird. Save the exciting stuff, and learn who you can trust. The lionesses will want to get to know you, but let them make those moves. It adds some mystery and likability to you.

The fifth rule is an easy one because being a man automatically gets you points among most of the female staff. Congrats! You've passed rule 5. I don't care what you think, men bring a different dynamic to the workplace. Not saying better or worse — just different. Our dynamic works wonderfully mixed with the female staff. They like working with men.

My friend's wife is the nurse manager of an ICU. When I told her about this book, she said in a playful, but frustrated tone, "Men in nursing are so spoiled. I was passed up for a promotion because my competition was a guy. I was more qualified and had more experience, and he beat me. He got the promotion! His resume was that he was a dude!" All I could do was laugh because I knew it was true. She then exclaimed, "I am just as guilty, though, because I always hire men. If I interview a guy, I'm going to hire him. It's just how it is. We love working with men." We have a special advantage in this profession. Play your cards right and enjoy the perks!

KING OF THE JUNGLE

You can thrive as a male nurse in the jungle. You can have it where the lionesses jump to help you or even do some of your work for you. They will work hard to make sure you are happy and having a great shift. Here is how you become a king of the jungle.

King status is not easy, and it can take years to perfect. Being king doesn't mean you rule the jungle. It means that the lionesses love you and take great care of you. The first rule of king status is never to brag about king status. It will make the lionesses want to bring you back to reality. The second rule of king status is that the lionesses rule the jungle. They can make you prey quickly if you mess up. Always work to keep them happy.

I met my wife, Jessica, working night shifts on a small psychiatric floor. We worked twelve-hour night shifts together. She is an amazing psych nurse and would end up doing a lot of my work for me. I bragged about this when we were dating. "You couldn't help my charm and did all my work." She laughed and said, "I knew exactly what you were doing, but I still chose to do your work anyway." I told her, "That is mastery!"

It takes time to become a king. You cannot walk onto a unit and expect it to happen right away. Like I said earlier, they will eat you alive. It takes working with these nurses to get to a point where they like you, trust you, respect you, and love working with you. This book will teach you all my secrets on being a king of the jungle.

Here's more about the types of lionesses you'll encounter throughout your career.

THE NINE TYPES OF LIONESSES

1. **Alpha lioness.** The mama lioness takes care of the unit. She is in charge a lot and takes care of the other nurses like they are her cubs.

2. **Perfect nurse.** She loves nursing; it's her calling. She works really hard at her job, and she is always positive.

3. **Complainer.** She is pissed off a lot, complains about everything, and loves the gossip. She wants to quit but never will.

4. **Know-it-all.** She is not always the best nurse, but she acts like she knows everything. She asks a lot of questions during report to sound smart, and she can be kind of annoying.

5. **Always drowning/busy.** She means well, but she is always running around, behind on her work, and she cannot prioritize her days.

6. **Unreliable.** She calls off often, shows up late a lot, and is never sure if she did everything she was supposed to on her shift. You end up fixing a lot of her mistakes.

7. **Baby nurse.** She is the new nurse — timid, still learning, worried about calling doctors, and worried if she is doing things correctly.

8. **Chill nurse.** She is laid-back and doesn't get worked up about too much. That doesn't mean she isn't good at her job; some chill nurses are in fact the best nurses. They just don't care about the small, unimportant things others stress about.

9. **Old crotchety.** She has been a nurse for a long time, and she does not care about the small nuances of nursing. She

is either quiet or very outspoken. She is a wealth of knowledge and great to learn from. She can also be scary and intimidating. She loves burning a doctor or nurse who thinks they are hot shit.

You want these lionesses to be your allies on this crazy career path. By the end of this book, you will know how to work and flourish among them. Let's start from the beginning. Welcome to the jungle!

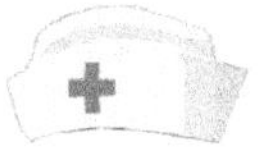

Chapter 2

Nursing School

"How many nurses does it take to screw in a light bulb?
None; it's delegated to the nursing student." — Unknown

IF YOU ARE ENTERING NURSING SCHOOL OR LOOKING TO become a male nurse, this chapter is for you. If you are already a nurse, then I hope you get a good chuckle out of this chapter. You are a survivor.

The obvious first step to becoming a male nurse is going to nursing school. Nursing school is more about survival than anything. The men with the ability to keep their heads down and do the work graduate.

Nursing was created by women, and this is their education program. In my program, the sciences were easy because there was only one correct answer on the test. As a man, I like having one correct answer. When you get into nursing school, that all changes. Women created nursing exams. They give you two correct answers, and whichever answer you pick . . . you are wrong. You must choose the answer that is "most correct."

Here's an example:

You find that a patient is blue and having difficulty breathing. What do you do?

    a. Check oxygenation level

    b. Check respiratory rate

    c. Ask, "Are you feeling OK?"

    d. Check responsiveness

You would do all four interventions. But which one do you do *first*? We do some of them at the same time. Pick the "most correct answer." Your thought process would look something like . . .

"OK, I would definitely check their oxygenation level, but respiratory rate is important as well. I would ask them, 'Are you feeling OK?' but if they are not responsive, then we have a big problem on our hands. Ahhh . . ."

Some of you are wondering what the correct answer is. All four answers — a, b, c, and d — are correct. When you are a nurse, you do all of these at the same time. This is exactly the kind of question you will see as a nursing student. Pick the most correct answer. Excited for school?

There were so many debates held in class where the teacher would even agree with the students. She would say, "Yes, that was the correct answer, but the most correct answer is ______ because that's what my book says."

Nursing school: where there are two right answers, and whichever you choose is the wrong answer.

Most states have decided to make nursing school too expensive, exceedingly difficult to get into, and hard to pass. They added extra rules, wait times, and classes that do not contribute to being a nurse. It is ridiculous. Would it not be more beneficial to get nurses into the profession simpler and quicker? Would that help the nationwide nursing shortage? I know; it makes too much sense. I digress since I do not run this show, but choosing a school can be a daunting task.

My advice will always be to choose the cheapest and fastest path, and then just get through it. I received my diploma in a twenty-two-month accelerated course, and I got my bachelor's degree online. My hospital paid for my education, and I am so happy I did it this way. I would choose it every time.

After you get your registered nursing degree, no one is trying to fail you anymore. It was mostly, "Here's tens of thousands of dollars. Thank you for the piece of paper." Bachelor's of nursing . . . woo! It didn't change anything about how I care for patients, but some of you will need it to accelerate your career path. If you are going to get your bachelor's degree, then it is easier to do it right away after you get your license. It's easier when you are mentally in school mode to continue forward. It's more difficult to stop and start up again later, but nurses succeed both ways. Just remember that it is harder to be motivated later. If you think you need it, then go get it.

My wife took the traditional four-year college approach to nursing. She will tell you the exact same thing I am telling you now. Get it done as fast and cheap as possible. She went to a very good college and came out with a bachelor's of science in nursing. She also came out with over $100,000 in student loan debt.

Nurses do not make enough money to pay top dollar for school. You can look at the student loan debt disaster in this country. It is disgusting what they do to young people financially, but that is a subject for another book. This is about putting you on the best path for your nursing career. Trust me and go the cheap route because it gets you to the same place. Luckily, my wife worked for an in-need hospital, and the government was willing to pay half of her debt down for her in exchange for two years of work. Seek out all the ways to pay for your schooling and avoid loans whenever possible.

Make sure to look for scholarships for men in nursing. Men are in high demand: take advantage of that. A quick internet search turned up multiple scholarship opportunities for nurses — specifically men in nursing. I am not going to include a list here because it could change in the future. Make sure to find and apply for these scholarships. Take advantage of being a man going to nursing school.

There is a real fear when you graduate that you don't really know what you are doing. I know I felt this way. It can be scary and overwhelming when you get your first job. I will tell you that it is OK because you are not alone. The good news is that you will learn most of "how to be a nurse" once you get your job (that is, unless you have been a CNA or nursing assistant in the past and know a little bit of the nursing game). Still, do not stress when you get out of nursing school. If you are at a good hospital and nursing unit, they will fill in the gaps and teach you the ropes.

Most of nursing school survival is persistence. It is having the mindset that you are going to make it, no matter what. Your tenacity will be tested time and again. Stay persistent, and know that dumber people than you have graduated and become nurses.

You now have the survival skills to make it through nursing school and become a real-life male nurse. Congratulations, Focker! Now it's time to get a job. Let's check out the many nursing specialties out there.

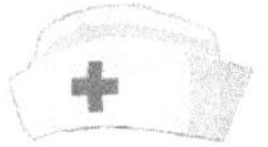

The Job

"Gotta pass the pills to pay the bills." — Unknown

A GIANT PERK OF NURSING IS THAT THERE ARE SO MANY opportunities within our profession. There are a multitude of diverse specialties. You can learn and grow through this profession, and there really is something for everyone. Nursing gives you the flexibility to pivot and move throughout your career.

A key survival tip is to never feel stuck where you are. There is power in that, and it's another huge perk of our profession. Some specialties pay very well, while others may come with better hours or benefits. It all depends on the amount of schooling you want to complete and where you want to go career-wise. It is good to get a plan together from the beginning, especially if you want to get into the upper echelon of nursing and be a nurse anesthetist or a flight nurse.

A common misconception is that after nursing school you should do medical-surgical nursing for a year before going to an advanced unit like the ICU or ED. This is false. I put this in my book because I have heard this lie told too often. The ICU, ED, OR, telemetry, etc. will train you to work in that specialty. Specialties require different types of nursing skills than medical-surgical nursing, and you don't need experience first. I love medical-surgical nursing, so I am not talking smack on it. I worked in medical-surgical units for a huge chunk of my career. If you want to do a specialty in nursing, just go do it!

Popular Nursing Specialties

Medical-surgical	PACU
Telemetry	ED
ICU	Oncology
Intermediate care unit	Flight
Psychiatric/behavioral health	Pediatric
Orthopedics	Anesthesia
Travel	Physician's assistant
Nurse manager	Nurse practitioner
Nurse supervisor	Labor and delivery
Administration (CNO)	Midwife
Operating room	Wound care nurse
Education	Nurse consultant
Doctor's office	Public/private school
Case management	Hospice
Medical/pharmaceutical sales	Public health
	Military
Dialysis	Rehab/long-term
Nursing home	acute care

There are very happy people in every one of these positions. Hopefully this helps you understand the opportunity out there for you as a male nurse. I suggest that if there is something on this list you are interested in, finding someone who is working that job and ask them for advice. They usually can give you the best path forward and save you a ton of time. Just knowing the right person will get you where you want to go much faster.

There also are a lot of areas for growth or movement. Sometimes we go down one path in nursing to transition later to a specialty we really love. You can see from my work history that this profession can take you many places. It is one of the best parts about nursing — mobility.

Now that we have a job, what's next? For your survival orientation, I'm going to show you the key survival technique that has defined my career as a nurse.

Chapter 4

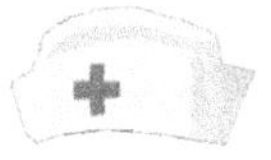

I Really Like That Guy!

"Charisma is the perfect blend of warmth and confidence."
— *Vanessa Van Edwards*

NOW IT'S TIME TO GET INTO THE NITTY GRITTY OF MALE nurse survival. This book isn't about how to chart or pass medications; you learn all that in school and orientation to your unit. This book is about what they don't teach you — how to survive and thrive as a nurse. It answers questions that you might not fully appreciate when you start your nursing career but become very important later: How do you get the best shifts? How do you get the time off you want? How do you get the best patients? How do you achieve better patient satisfaction? How do you solidify that yearly raise?

It all begins with whether they *like* you.

I am assuming that you will do good work because being good at your job is important. You must strive to be a good nurse. People won't like you if you are terrible at the fundamentals of nursing. Obviously, you have to be competent at your job and do your work correctly. That is a given.

Being likable and charismatic gets you all the added perks to really win. A big reason why I have been successful in my nursing career is because I am a likable guy. It sounds superficial, but it's the truth. Need a shift covered? No problem! Time off? Have it! Great review that gets a raise? Of course! Being liked is a key to survival.

We all want to work with people we like, know, and trust. We want to be around people who make us feel comfortable. You must have good character. Character means that you are a good person and mean well. If you are manipulative, then people will eventually figure it out. Charisma, character, and a good attitude will take you far in this profession. Being well-liked will help you get a better work environment, better assignments, approved time off requests, extra help during your shift, and more. Can you be a miserable, unlikable guy and still be a nurse? Of course! I have met many miserable, unlikable nurses. They struggle more and have a harder time. If you are miserable, then your shifts and your nursing life will be miserable too. Choose to be likable and make your life — and the lives of everyone else — a little better.

The only thing you can control in this world is your attitude. I don't remember where I heard this advice, but it always stuck with me. Pause and think about it for a second. You can't control the administration, the workload, the patients, or your team, but you can control your attitude toward it all. Some people don't want to hear or believe this, but it is true. You have the choice to bring a great and helpful attitude to work with you. You can decide the version of you who shows up to work every day. Have a great attitude and the other nurses will love working with you.

TOP PEOPLE YOU WANT TO LIKE YOU

1. **Your manager.** Managers give you raises, approve your time off, and more.

2. **Scheduler.** To me, the scheduler is one of the most important roles. Time is your most precious commodity. You want the scheduler to like you and work with you so you can get the schedule you want.

3. **Charge nurses.** You want the good assignments with the good patients. You don't want the hard patients all the time. If the charge nurses like you, they take care of you. If they don't like you, then they can make your shifts more difficult.

4. **Nursing team.** They will jump in and help you, pick up a shift for you, and cover for you if you make a mistake. Getting along with the nursing team also creates a more enjoyable work environment.

5. **CNAs.** They will make sure to get all the stuff you need and that your patients are taken care of. They make your shift smoother and back you up when you need them. They will even do extra work at times just for you.

6. **Doctors.** If they like and trust you, it is easier to get what you need from them. No one likes talking to doctors with bad attitudes. If they like you, they will be nicer to you. They will also let you off the hook if you forget something or make a mistake.

7. **Patients.** If they like you, then they will have a better hospital experience. Being likable helps the patient trust you. If they trust you, then you are able to care for them better and they are happier. A happy patient makes for happy nurses. They will let you slide if you make a mistake and usually be less needy. They also give you the benefit of the doubt if you forget something.

BEING LIKED BY YOUR MANAGER

I found the key to being liked by your manager is quite simple: show up on time, do your job, and don't complain. Sounds easy, but many nurses screw this up. Be polite and respectful to them, and they should be respectful to you. If you are in good spirits when you converse with them, then they will feel good about having you on the team. Pick up an extra shift or come in early to help them for some bonus points.

In my first job as a nurse, I was devastated to learn that it was hospital policy that nurses work every other weekend. This was fine in the summer, but in the winter my family and best friends all went to the local ski resort. My absolute favorite thing to do was snowboard and hang out with my friends on the weekends. I was only twenty years old and at the time sponsored by a snowboard shop. This was all being ruined by my new nursing career. I knew I would be miserable on the weekends working while everyone I knew was having a blast at the slopes.

I was working only a few months when I approached my unit manager about my dilemma. My boss, Diane, liked me because of all the techniques I am teaching you here. I wasn't necessarily aware of them at the time, but they worked out hugely in my favor. I told her my weekend dilemma, and she said, "We can work something out." She ended up giving me a Monday, Tuesday, Wednesday set schedule through the winter so I could snowboard and hang with my friends all weekend. I was able to spend every Thursday through Sunday at the ski resort, and it was amazing. I could not believe I got every weekend off! It still astonishes me and fills me with gratitude today. Do you think

I worked hard for Diane and had her back forever after that? Absolutely!

My mom couldn't believe it when I told her. She said, "You are so unbelievably lucky. How did you pull that off?" My mom was a nurse for twenty years, and she knows how hospitals work. New nurses do not get weekends off. I told her my boss just likes me and is awesome! After winter, I approached Diane and asked what I could do to help out, and I worked every Sunday night through the summer and fall for her. It didn't bother me; my Sunday nights were easy. I would have done anything for Diane, and she is still to this day one of my favorite managers of all time. I am glad she liked me!

BEING LIKED BY THE SCHEDULER

You want to treat the scheduling person very well so they give you the shifts you want. Be polite and respectful by saying "please" and "thank you." Work with them, and they will usually work with you. They have shifts that they need filled; pick up a hole for them every once in a while. Figure out where they have needs and see if you can work with that schedule. If you help them, they will usually be willing to adjust to help you. Soon, you can have the dream schedule that fits your life.

BEING LIKED BY THE NURSING STAFF AND CNAS

The first step is to smile and be welcoming. People like to be around happy people. Even if you are mad that you had to come to work, try not to show it.

Be a helpful nurse. We are all a team and need each other. Be willing and able for a quick boost up in bed or to waste a narcotic. If you are there to make their shift easier, then they will love you for it. No one is above basic patient care. I see nurses who believe this, though. Help your CNAs and techs because they work hard and we are all in it together. Jump in to help in these simple situations and other nurses will jump and help you when you need it.

Don't bitch and complain. Nursing can suck enough without working with miserable people. Try and make the best of it. If you are enjoyable to work with, then it can be a good shift no matter what happens. You want to be the guy other nurses are excited to work with. If they know it will be a good shift with you, then you will be the favorite nurse.

Do the little things. Answer a call bell on someone who isn't your patient, help a patient who isn't yours to the bathroom, or pass a pain medication for another nurse. Sometimes it just takes asking, "Do you need help with anything?" Most of the time they will say, "No, I'm OK," but it lets them know that you are there if they need you. You get credit just for asking. This is an important tip. Do this for your nurses and your nursing assistants. These little things make an impact. You don't have to always be running around doing other people's work, but once in a while makes a big difference.

Make sure you are an easy nurse to give and receive report from. Be respectful of the other nurses' time. Be someone who shows up on time, gets report quickly, and gets the other nurse out on time (bonus points if you get them out early). There is nothing that drives nurses crazier than getting out late because the other nurse takes their sweet time or shows up late. Don't ask too many questions during report. Make sure you get the important stuff; the rest is in the computer. There is plenty of time to look something up or read a full history if you must know it. You don't need to hold up report for unimportant details that you can find in the computer. Let them give you the important things and go home. It makes them much happier — and you more likable.

Don't ever make the nurses or doctors feel dumb. I see nurses who ask questions just to make themselves feel smart, or try to catch the other nurse off guard. Make others feel good. If they don't know an answer, tell them, "No problem, I will figure it out." If you are nice about it, they will usually come back to you with the answer.

Don't make stuff up during report or lie. I found that a good "I don't know" is better than making something up. If it is important information, then go find it for them. If the information isn't important, then let them figure it out. Some nurses love to know everything about a patient, including all the unimportant details. Everyone has their own style; just be honest with your team. If you don't know the answer, tell them that. If the information isn't important, let them know where they can look for the answer.

There will be times when people want to teach you things, or tell you how to do things you already know. This happens a lot, and it usually comes from a good place. They are trying to be helpful. I recommend, even if you know the information, to be polite, listen, and even play along. This will give them the satisfaction that they helped, and it doesn't hurt one bit in the long run. If you are rude, cut them off, or tell them you already know this information, it could hurt their feelings or make you appear unteachable. I find it much easier and smoother to listen and say, "Sounds good, thank you." This may sound unusual reading it now, but I can't tell you how many times people try to teach me things that I have done for years, especially as a travel nurse. The simple phrase "sounds good, thank you" is more charming and swift than explaining that you already know all this information.

Here's an example:

> **The patient is having chest pain.**
>
> **The charge nurse calls over to me,**
> **"You should call the doctor and get an EKG**
> **and cardiac labs."**
>
> **Me: "Sounds good, thank you."**
>
> ***This is so much better than "No shit!"***

BEING LIKED BY DOCTORS

Doctors are another group of peers we have a lot of contact with. I always recommend getting along with your providers. Doctors will also ask you to do things, maybe even after you have already done them. I am always polite, respond with simple answers, and usually say "sounds good" just like before.

Calling doctors is usually the scariest thing to do for a new nurse. When calling or communicating needs to them, keep it short, sweet, and precise. I found that the more direct and simple the message was, the easier it was to get what I needed and get off the phone. Doctors like this because it looks like you know your stuff and you don't waste their time. They are busy, and it is important to respect that. Don't drone on and on about your patient. Just give them the information they need to make a decision. It's simple.

> **"Hey Dr. Howser, it's Chris on 5 West. I have your patient Bruce Wayne, and he is having chest pain. He has a history of chest pain, his vital signs are stable, and he isn't in any distress. I put him on telemetry and was going to order an EKG and some cardiac labs. Is there anything else you think we might need?"**

Now, I might have more information than in this example, but you get the picture. If I have a good relationship with the doctor, they will trust me and my judgment. I believe in keeping it concise, as providers have a lot of patients but not a lot of patience.

BEING LIKED BY YOUR PATIENTS

Say "hello" and introduce yourself when you first meet them. Smile and be welcoming. Let them know that you see them as a person, not just another patient, and that you are a person too.

Before leaving the room, I like to ask patients if they need anything else and tell them I will be back. Reassurance is important. It acknowledges that you are here to help. Referencing their medications times is good, too, so they know their schedule. I will always let them know to call me if they need anything. This builds a good relationship from the start.

Work hard to do exactly what you tell them you are going to do. If you tell them you will be back in an hour with their pain medications, then do it. You won't be perfect all the time, but a good "I'm so sorry I got caught up" will bring forgiveness.

<table>
<tr><td align="center">TIP:</td></tr>
<tr><td>If you are late with a medication, water, or anything the patient requested, make sure to be in a hurry when you bring it into the room. Be the nurse rushing into the room, apologizing and working fast to get it to them. Be working quickly to fix the mistake. This nonverbally signals that you were rushing around and got in there as fast as you could. Even if you were sitting around playing on the computer and completely forgot, you remain likable because you were rushed and concerned about getting their needs met. It's a simple tip, but this will keep you in good graces with your patients when you mess up.</td></tr>
</table>

DON'T COMPLAIN

This is a tough one. We all need to let off some steam from time to time. It is best that if you do complain that you try to make it constructive. It is seductive to be drawn into the negativity. You will be around other people who love to complain — even thrive on it. Try to avoid this. It will make you unhappy at your job, and you do not want the reputation. There are always going to be problems and scenarios that annoy you. There is a lot of it in this profession. Really try to be constructive with your criticism. Attempt to make your unit and shift better, but don't get caught in the trap of just complaining.

Find a venting partner. I am lucky that my wife and mother are nurses, so I can vent to them after a bad shift. It can be difficult if your partner is not in health care to understand or relate. It might be helpful to keep up with a nurse who you went to school with or to have someone you can call and complain to. I would recommend not venting to anyone you work with unless you trust them 100 percent. It can come back to bite you.

WHEN TO BE UNLIKABLE

There will be times you absolutely will want to stand up for yourself. Being likable should never go against your values or patient safety or put your job at risk. You have to be respected as a nurse. Do not let people walk all over you. A confident and direct "no" is great when you need to use it.

I believe time is a top priority. I have worked places that believe that their nurses are indentured servants. They refuse time off, create scheduling conflicts, and break promises. This drives me crazy. It is understandable that they cannot accommodate every request for every employee, but if you are working within the agreed parameters, then hold your ground and make sure you get your time off.

When the coronavirus pandemic was just starting, many hospitals were trying to figure out their action plans. The hospital I was working at had a low census at this point and no emergency status. I overheard a respiratory therapist telling the other staff that the hospital might not let her take her time off just in case there was a spike in patients. This was approved time off she planned months ago. The hospital was slow, and she was asking the other staff members' advice on what to do. My response was, "Hey, this isn't Russia. They don't own you. Go on vacation." This may sound a little over the top, but I assure you that for some hospitals, it is exactly how they treat you: "We need you more than your family." Don't allow this to happen to you.

Remember, you agreed to this job in exchange for its benefits. Those benefits include breaks, vacations, and sick days. Don't kill yourself for a job that would replace you in a heartbeat if you left.

The unit never fell apart because I took my approved time off. If I needed time for family, vacation, or just to have time off, it was always my top priority. The best part about nursing is that we are in high demand. I have seen people give up so much for a nursing unit that treated them terribly later. Guess what? If you died tomorrow, they would replace you or have your team run short. It is the truth. I am not saying burn your team or manager by running them short or leaving them hanging, but take your time off.

New nurses are a little different story. New nurses have to pay their dues. The new nurses usually get last pick for time off and scheduling. This is just the nature of the game. If you are new, please be smart and don't come in trying to overthrow the senior staff. They will eat you. The senior nurses paid their dues and deserve to be a priority. If you have a good manager that is fair, then usually they will work with you the best they can. I got lucky with the nurses at my first job. If they like you, then this is much easier to accomplish.

If your manager is an unfair jerk, then moving on to a new job or separate unit can be the right choice. Your manager, hospital, and unit do not own you. Have a mindset of, "I can always get another job. I am great at what I do, and somewhere else would love to have me." This keeps you out of a scarcity mindset and allows you to make decisions that aren't driven by emotions. Never forget that you deserve respect wherever you work. When you finish this book, you will have all the skills to be in high demand.

Now that you are liked and respected by the people around you, how do you survive when things get crazy? How do you survive the chaos?

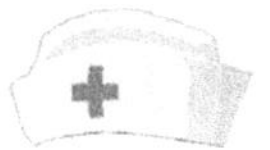

Chapter 5

Can I Speak to Your Time Manager?

"Either run the day, or the day runs you." — Jim Rohn

NURSING IS STRUCTURED CHAOS. YOUR DAY CAN QUICKLY turn into disaster. It can also go smooth as silk. The problem is that you never know which day you are going to have. There are times I envy an office worker with the same mundane routine every day. Your day is boring? I am freaking jealous. I don't know if it is my day to get pooped on, have a patient die, or have a doctor decide it's time to do those fifteen tests and procedures on my shift.

The day will start one way and can take a drastic turn quickly. There's only so much routine. And you can only comment on the easiness of a shift after it is done. Don't you dare say, "It's quiet." You will get clawed to death as it turns into a disaster. It will get busy, and when you think it can't get any worse, it does! The way you manage your time is extremely important for success and survival.

Time management is a top skill to learn as a nurse. Prioritizing your day takes practice. Each unit runs differently, as does each specialty. The ED's flow is much different than an OR or medical floor, but good time management principles carry over everywhere. Whether your day starts out fast or you build into the excitement, you need to know how to prioritize and manage your time. The hours are going to pass either way; the better you manage your workload, the better the day goes. This ultimately comes with experience, but there are nurses who have been working for years and still can't seem to figure this out. It is worth your time and energy to get good at this skill. Practice it and prioritize.

How do you get better at managing your time? I will share some simple principles that have helped me over the years. I believe that how you start your day is how you win the day! The beginning of your shift has a large effect on how the rest of your shift turns out. If you want better days, then you need to have a strong start to the day.

My goal at the start of my shift is to always get report quickly and get organized quickly. I don't even believe in coming in early to get organized, but some nurses do. I get to work on time and jump right into report to get the other shift out fast. Some nurses I watch take a ton of time getting started. They get a long report, then they go get breakfast or coffee, then they sit down and take their time looking at their charts and getting organized. It starts their shift out slow and potentially running away from them. It doesn't matter if it is my third shift in a row and I know my patients and what the shift will look like: I still get report and organized first thing, and I do it fast. I know there are no guarantees and that the day can change in an instant.

Once I am organized, I know if anyone needs medications or interventions first thing in the morning. Call bells could start and doctors could come rounding, so being organized quickly lets you be ready for whatever the day throws at you.

My next goal is to get my assessments completed and charted as soon as possible. Grouping your cares together is a key skill to learn. If someone needs a medication first thing in the morning, then that will be my first assessment. Depending on my assignment, I will assess all my patients and then chart on all of them right away. If it is busy, I will try to get half of my charting done because then I only have to finish the other half later. Charting is a time-consuming task, so it's good to get a few done and break it up. Then I go do my other interventions and assessments and chart those next.

It is a relief to know that your charting is taken care of early in the shift. I watch nurses put charting off until later in the day. They dread doing it, procrastinate, and pay the price. Then the busy part of the shift happens like it always does, and they are stressed. They can't even remember what they did eight hours ago at the beginning of their shift. This then leads to more stress, less productivity, and, many times, leaving late to go home.

Medication administration is my other top goal. There are usually scheduled medications early in the shift. I start passing medications as soon as possible within the scheduled medication timeframe. I know that if I get my patients assessed, charting completed, and medications passed early in my shift, then I am ready for whatever is thrown at me. I attribute this plan to much of my success. I always get out on time at the end of my shift. Ninety-nine percent of the time, if I get out late, it is because I am waiting on the incoming shift to give report and they are taking too long. If you follow my strategies, then you will almost always be out on time too. Starting your shift strong will lead to more good days.

You may be thinking, "That's great, but my specialty doesn't run like that." That is true; the way I do things may not work for you or your specialty. So, how do I teach you if every unit is different? How can you learn if your specialty or unit runs differently? Simple! Find the nurse who gets out on time and gets the job done on time. Find the nurse who has more good days than bad days. Find the nurse who is the least stressed on the unit. Ask that nurse for advice. Ask them how they plan their day. Ask them how they are able to float by while others are drowning.

If you don't want to ask them for advice, simply observe them throughout their day. Watch how they start their day, prioritize their tasks, and handle situations. You can learn a lot by observation. If you want the crash course, then just ask to follow them. Tell them you want to learn how they manage their time and prioritize their shift. I bet they'll show you exactly how they organize and run their day. I bet they know a few shortcuts too. And I didn't say to ask the charge nurse or most passionate nurse. Find the nurse who has less stress and gets their work done on time. That is the nurse you want to learn a thing or two from.

If you manage your time well, you will be more likable. No one wants to follow a nurse who can't get their work done on time. They want to work with nurses who get their tasks completed when they are supposed to. Your nurses will be happier because you have more time to help them. Your doctors will be happy because their orders are getting done when they need them. Your patients will be happy because they are getting what they need when they need it. Make prioritizing a priority. Every unit is different, but work on your time management for long-term success as a nurse.

Now, how do we use that time more effectively? How do we maximize our efforts and the efforts of our team? Well, you need to ask for help!

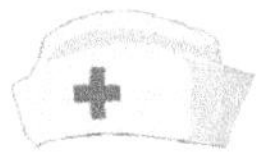

Chapter 6

Help Me!

*"What cruel mistakes are sometimes made by benevo-
lent men and women in matters of business about which
they can know nothing and think they know a great deal."*
—Florence Nightingale

THIS MAY BE THE *MOST IMPORTANT CHAPTER* IN THIS
entire book. If I had to pick the greatest weapon for your survival as a male nurse it is . . . *ask for help!*

It doesn't matter how long you have been a nurse. There
will always be things you don't know. The worst nursing trait
is to think you know everything. Don't ever be scared to ask for
help. This is especially true as a male nurse because the female
nurses will be open to helping you. Even if I think I know what
I'm supposed to do, I might still ask for clarification just to be
sure. It is better to ask for help than make a mistake that hurts
someone or your nursing career.

"Are these drugs compatible?"

"How do I order this?"

"Which doctor do I call?"

"How do I do this procedure? Can you show me?"

**"Is there anything I have to do to get the patient ready
for this procedure?"**

Never be afraid to ask for help. If you follow my survival instructions on being likable, then you can get away with asking just about anything.

Most mistakes I see nurses make happen when they didn't ask for help when they should have. As men, we are often taught that asking for help can be a sign of weakness. We may even try and save face by acting like we know, even though we really don't. Ever hear that men won't ask for directions when they are lost? That doesn't work in nursing. I promise that asking for help will be your greatest strength. When you are willing to ask for help, it shows that you are confident in yourself and that you want to do the best for your patients. You care more about your patients than your ego. It will be key to a long and strong career.

If you are likable, there is a very good possibility that the nurses will make your life a whole lot easier. They may even jump in and do tasks and cares for you. Need an IV replaced? There is a good chance that nurse who is good at IVs will do it if she likes you and you ask politely. Need a medication passed while you are a little busy? I bet that charge nurse will help if you say "please."

Make sure to show a lot of gratitude when someone helps you. I recommend above average gratitude. This will ensure that they help you again next time.

> **"Thank you so much for placing that IV! You made my day so much better."**
>
> **"You are the best!"**

Gratitude is the essential element. It is scientifically proven that people are happier when they perform an act of kindness or help someone else. In a way, you are helping them as much as they are helping you.

> **"Performing random acts of kindness helps boost your psychological health by activating the release of dopamine, the feel-good neurotransmitter in the brain, often referred to as a 'helper's high.' This is based on the theory that giving produces endorphins in the brain that mimic a morphine high.[2]"**

You are making the other nurses healthier and happier by allowing them to help you. It's science!

Asking for help is so important. It's a lesson I try to teach to my students, when I have them. One day on a travel assignment, I was the only other nurse there to help teach students. I was honestly a little nervous. I had not taught a student in a long time, and I was worried I might ruin them.

As I was trying to impart my eternal wisdom on this student, I remembered the most important lesson: even after fifteen years, you will never know everything. You have to learn the basics and learn to do them well. You then use what you've got when you've got it. We have to be creative. They are going to change the rules and policies on us constantly in this profession. The protocols are always changing and being tweaked. Do you know how many different ways they've found to do CPR

---

2 Lizette Borrelli, "Random Acts of Kindness Raise Dopamine Levels and Boost Your Mood," Medical Daily, April 26, 2016, https://www.medicaldaily.com/random-acts-kindness-sweet-emotion-helping-others-dopamine-levels-383563.

over the past fifteen years? Hell, different hospitals have different protocols for the same procedures. The important thing is that you perform the basics correctly and ask for help when you need it.

WHEN ASKING FOR HELP GOES WRONG

I had never seen Walt so flustered. He is a great nurse, and he was normally very calm and collected. But this night, he was completely distraught. It was concerning to me. I was getting report from him and began to learn about what had taken place a few hours earlier. If it happened to me, I would have completely quit nursing.

Walt received a TURP from the OR a few hours prior to me coming on shift. A TURP is a transurethral resection of the prostate — a surgery to remove parts of the prostate gland through the penis. As a guy, it sounds worse than it is, but there is no incision needed. They just go up through the urethra. For us as the nurse, it is usually a moderate to easy patient assignment. The worst part is the catheter and the continuous bladder irrigation system. Because you just chopped up the prostate, the urine is bloody and clotted. You must keep the catheter from clotting by running large bags of normal saline that flush the catheter. This keeps everything moving. You go through the saline bags rather quickly, and the urine bag then fills up fast. You do this until the urine clears up and the prostate heals. The most difficult work is maintaining the hanging bangs and emptying the bloody urine.

Walt was having a hell of a time with the catheter and irrigation system on this TURP patient. The catheter kept clotting off. He was manually flushing it, maneuvering the catheter, and trying everything in his nursing arsenal to get it all working. It just kept clotting on him. He asked a fellow nurse if she could assist him on completely changing out the catheter system. This should have been just a routine catheter change, and hopefully the new system would work appropriately.

Walt removed the old catheter and inserted the new one, just like he had done many times before. Men are not difficult to catheterize because you can easily see the hole. The new catheter was inserted and started to flow beautifully, but then all of a sudden, it stopped again. Sweaty and frustrated, Walt began another attempt at manually flushing this new catheter.

These are situations that they don't prepare you for — not how to flush a catheter, but what comes next. Walt proceeded to take his syringe and saline and try to open up the catheter again. He was beyond frustrated and really tried to force the liquid in. What Walt wasn't expecting was the explosion that came back out of the tube. It came out with so much force past him — like a cannon! — and by instinct he moved to the side. Luck would have it that the bloody urine missed him completely. The problem was that Nicole, his nurse helper, was right behind him. Walt turned to see the nurse who took the time out of her day to assist him covered from head to toe with bloody, clotted urine.

Walt was in shock. Nicole just walked out of the room and down the hallway. Another nurse spotted her and said it looked like the scene from the movie *Carrie* where she gets pig blood dumped on her. She was just walking down the hall covered in bloody piss. The nurse grabbed her, and luckily there was an empty patient room close by. She took her directly to the shower to hose off. Everyone was happy there weren't any patients or family members around to see a nurse walking down the hall like that. Talk about an experience.

When I arrived to work a few hours later, Walt was still in a bit of shock. He managed to get the catheter working, but he was still flabbergasted about the whole event. Nicole was actually still there finishing her shift in scrubs she borrowed from the OR. She was in really good spirits about the whole thing. Walt felt awful. The good news was the patient was fine and free of any blood diseases. This was great news for Nicole, because she got some in her mouth too . . . ew!

I couldn't believe Nicole was still at work when I arrived. Like I said, I think I would have just left that day and never returned to nursing. The moral of the story is that help sometimes comes at a cost. The other moral is don't stand in the line of fire when someone is flushing a catheter. Nicole learned this the hard way. I want to ask anyone with an office job about their worst day of work ever. I bet a million dollars they can't beat Nicole!

This story is a wild and rare example where asking for help goes wrong. You should ask for help — and always be open to receiving it. Your long-term success and survival really depends on it. Nursing is a complex profession, and it is impossible to know everything. You don't want to live with the regret of a mistake that could have been prevented simply by asking for help. We all need help sometimes.

Now that you know how to ask for help, what do you do when shit hits the fan? As a nurse, this could literally happen to you.

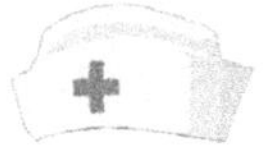

Chapter 7

Don't Panic

"Keep them alive until 7:05!" — Unknown

HAVE YOU EVER SAT AT YOUR JOB AND CONTEMPLATED your life's choices? It's early, you're tired, and now you're trying to decide why you did this to yourself? This was what I was going through one particular morning. I just finished report and sat down at the computer. I was preparing my day and looking through the electronic chart. I was not in a good mood, and I was tired. It looked like it was going to be a busy day, and I had some tough patients. I took a deep breath and thought to myself, "This day sucks."

I gazed downward to a small piece of paper taped to the bottom of the computer screen. A fortune cookie was taped there. It read, "Don't Panic." It caught me by surprise, and I instantly chuckled. It was perfect timing. This note changed my whole outlook, and I had a great day. It became the title of this chapter. It is essential advice for any nurse.

You want to be the rock in the chaos. You want to be the guy other nurses can lean on no matter what is happening. Be the guy who makes any shift go smoother and you will be loved by your team. You need to be the calm in the storm. You don't have to have all the answers, but you want to be the nurse who doesn't freak out when things are crazy. And they will get crazy!

If you are the strong nurse who doesn't panic, then the staff will enjoy working with you. They know it will be a good shift. There will be patients crashing, doctors writing orders, phones ringing, call bells dinging, and work to be done. It will be stressful. It is OK to take a moment here or there to be stressed, but around your coworkers, you need to be a rock.

I have seen a lot of nurses melt down when the pressure was on. It only makes them look unprofessional, and I never saw it help one bit. You want your team to feel confident they will survive — because you are there. They will trust you and love working with you.

This is a lesson imparted to me by a seasoned nurse at my first advanced cardiac life support (ACLS) class. You take this class if you are going to be working in some of the higher levels of nursing. It was at a big teaching hospital, and we had a big class. The nurse teaching the class had a fun and playful demeanor, and you knew she had seen a lot of chaos. She was set up in the front of the room with all her supplies and lifesaving gadgets. She had a dummy on the table hooked up for a demonstration. I was nervous because this was my first ACLS class and I didn't want to look like an idiot. I hoped she didn't call on me. This was serious, lifesaving education here.

I will never forget the instructor leaning over the dummy on the table and addressing the class. She had a defibrillator and monitor to simulate all the heart rhythms we may see. She could run a normal rhythm or any life-threatening scenario just with the push of a button. The first thing she did was set the rhythm on asystole — flatlining in the movies. This would be my nightmare as a nurse.

My first thought was, "Oh God, this is terrible!"

She looked up and calmly asked the class, "What heart rhythm is this?"

An ICU nurse in the corner said "asystole" out loud.

"Correct," the instructor said, and then asked, "What does this mean?"

Another student guessed, "We are in trouble?"

The instructor chuckled and said, "We aren't in trouble, but the patient is," with a smile.

Someone else said, "Their heart has stopped."

"Correct, and what does this mean?"

After a few seconds of quiet, she answered her own question: "They are dead!"

I ran the scenario in my head as if it were my patient and started to sweat. What would this be like? What would I do? Ahhh, my nightmare!

With a smile, the instructor put her arms up and in a loud and calm voice said, "Don't panic! It's OK. Don't freak out, because they are already dead. You can't screw up. They are dead. It's OK! Now let's see if we can bring them back to life."

I laughed because it caught me off guard . . . and I wasn't the only one either. The rest of the class smiled and laughed. "Don't panic. It's OK. They are already dead." It may sound bleak, but it was honest, and this immediately changed how I approached high-stress situations. "Don't panic" stuck with me all this time, even after this class. This silly interaction all those years ago taught me, "It's OK. Don't panic."

When we panic, we get into fight, flight, or freeze mode. Adrenaline starts pumping, we start thinking with our lizard brains, and we miss things. We are not as sharp as we should be. We miss things, we can't think clearly, and we are not able to make good decisions. If you remain calm, you can think clearly, evaluate the situation, and make the right decisions. It is imperative to survival.

Nursing is a high-stress profession. Stress is also the number one killer in the world. Stress is a causing factor to many of the ailments and diseases we see every day. As nurses, we are killing ourselves to save others. You want to live longer and be healthier? Work to keep your stress level down to a minimum. Having low stress may seem impossible in this profession, but when a stressful situation comes, remember: don't panic!

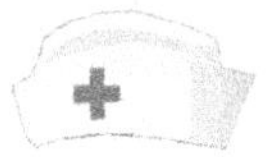

Day Shift versus Night Shift

"You don't truly know someone until you see what makes them die of laughter at 4 a.m." — Unknown

NURSING IS A TWENTY-FOUR-HOUR, SEVEN-DAY-A-WEEK JOB. It doesn't matter if it's a holiday or if the whole world is shut down. We still have to work. We may or may not even get to choose which shift we work. Some places make you rotate; with others, you may be able to pick your preference. I always liked working three twelve-hour shifts per week. Once you work eight hours, another four hours isn't bad. You get used to it, but there are so many different areas and shifts that may be available. Twelve-hour shifts are the most common, so I will talk about those here. You may see different start times depending on the hospital, which could include starting at 5:00 a.m., 6:00 a.m., or 7:00 a.m. Some places have shifts in the middle, like 11:00 a.m. to 11:00 p.m. I personally would never work somewhere that had a shift that started at 5:00 a.m., but some people like it. If you are new to nursing, it's good to know that we have to work off that lunch break. Make sure to add that thirty minutes on the end of a shift. I didn't know this when I started.

When you become a nurse, you get the privilege of working some crazy hours. Day shift and night shift have some similarities, but also some major differences. I remember my first night shift; I hated it. There is a reason they call it the "graveyard shift." I was up while everyone else was sleeping, and it was awful.

Then, I started to really like the flow of night shift, the crazy people I worked with, and being up while the sun was up before work. I worked night shifts for years.

Eventually, staying up all night really started to kick my butt, and I went back to day shifts. I got to really understand the differences between the two shifts again. It is also entertaining how both shifts complain about each other. I think it is just a lack of understanding of what each shift goes through. I thought it was worth noting in this book. Everyone has their own preferences. Here is the difference between days and nights and how to survive each.

DAY SHIFT

You wake up, start your day, and really don't have time to think about work. You get up, get ready, and go into work. You have less time to stress about your upcoming shift. You are waking up and going through the motions to get to work.

The best part is there are usually a lot of people around to help in all the different specialty areas. Transport teams, therapists, pharmacists, technicians, physicians, and supervisors — there are many hands around to help you. This is nice because it helps you get through how busy day shifts can be.

It is nice to have the extra support during the day, but there is also a lot happening. There are more procedures, interventions, and cares happening during your shift. It can really get busy. There are more family members around, and it can seem like patients are constantly being moved around or things are constantly happening. This shift requires a lot of organizational skills.

Doctors are around in person more often. You can ask questions and get the orders you need right there. This is nice, and they are awake and usually in better moods during the day. It is much more convenient to talk in person for orders or interventions.

Staff meetings and everything else are built around your schedules. Day shift gets the priority with meetings. Night shifters have to get up early (feeling like zombies) and make it work to be at these meetings. They don't have meetings at 2:00 a.m.

You get to keep a normal sleep schedule during work and on your days off. You can mingle with the living, as I like to call it. Your life doesn't suffer due to your sleep schedule.

The negative is that you have to be on your game. There are administrators and managers around, and they can catch you relaxing. Even when you are fully caught up on your work, you have to be careful. I always feel like someone is watching me when I have a little break in the action. You will have to be more sneaky with your downtime activities, like playing on your phone. It feels weird chilling when other peers and teammates are running around crazy.

Another negative is that depending on the time of year, you have to work when it's dark outside both when you drive in and out of work. You don't really get to see sunlight depending on the time of year. I think it can get a little depressing. It is hard not getting to be outside with the sun shining.

NIGHT SHIFT

You wake up in the afternoon and have time to dwell — and sometimes dread — going to work. You don't get up and run right to work most of the time. It is the feeling of, "Wow, what a nice day. Sucks I have to go to work tonight."

Your sleep schedule is completely screwed. Sometimes you don't know what day it is. You fall asleep at weird times. You're exhausted, foggy, loopy, and all the other things you can imagine. This is the hardest part of night shifts. It is proven that you actually shave years off your life working nights. Sometimes not being around all the managers and staff can be worth it, though.

You rely heavily on your team. The nurses and techs are your resources because they may be all you have. Need a CT scan? You are the transport team. Patient wants to take a walk? Well, you are physical therapy. Sometimes it is all hands on deck simply because that's all you've got.

You have to call doctors who are sleeping and can be cranky. Many times, the doctors aren't in the hospital, or the doctor on call doesn't really know your patients. Calling a doctor is many times a last resort because we don't want to deal with them in the middle of the night. I always try to navigate as many options as possible before I have to wake up a doctor.

But, you can push things off onto the day shift. There are times when stuff isn't that important in the middle of the night. There are certain cares or small events that you have day shift handle because they have the staff and the doctors are awake. Patient wants a stool softener at 2:00 a.m. that they refused earlier in the day? Guess what? You pass that off to day shift in report because we aren't calling a doctor at 2:00 a.m. for pooping pills.

The bonus is there are no managers or administrators around to bother you. It's awesome if you like your space and can enjoy the downtime. You are able to get away with reading, watching a movie, or catching up with your coworkers. I always felt that if I did my job well, then I deserved this downtime. You put your life span and sanity on the line working nights, so you deserve your downtime.

You will usually get shift differential, which means more money in your paycheck. This is nice because those extra dollars add up. You deserve it for working nights.

If you work nights, then you can accomplish your to-do list during the day when everyone else is working. You are out in the world with fewer people around. It is definitely a perk. Have to make a doctor's appointment? You can do it any day of the week. Want to hit up the mall? It's less busy on a Tuesday afternoon. You get your time during the day to do things. My personal favorite was when it was a powder day on the ski slopes. I would go out after my shift for a few hours in the morning, then go home and sleep before working my next night shift. You can give up a little sleep and accomplish tasks while the rest of the world is at their day job.

The night shift is usually busiest for the first four hours and then slows down. It's not like this everywhere all the time, but it tends to be the nighttime flow in most places. You start your shift running, but it slows down into the night. It's not always the case, but it's what we hope for. This is a little different than day shifts, which start slower and ramp up to a sprint.

You will learn all your coworkers' deepest, darkest secrets from around 2:00 a.m. to 5:00 a.m. Make sure that you are good at keeping secrets and not gossiping. You don't want to make any enemies.

Night shift nurses tend to be more laid-back. You have to be a little crazy to work night shifts. I can say that because I am one of those crazy nurses.

Bring snacks and food. There is a good chance you don't have cafeteria service. It is a very real thing to become ravenous at night and eat everything. I feel like a nurse werewolf sometimes devouring the drawer of saltines at the nurse's station. Be careful though: there is a reason night shifters tend to add on a few pounds when they start working this shift.

Your family or friends won't understand what you are going through working nights. They might tell you they understand, but they really don't unless they have done it themselves. They will wonder why you are tired all the time. They will call you in the middle of the day not realizing you're sleeping. They will ask questions like, "You just woke up?" in a judgmental way. It will take everything to refrain from punching them. I had to explain to family members that I went to bed at 8:30 a.m. and it is now 12:30 p.m. That is four hours of sleep. I then would ask, "How many hours of sleep did you get last night?"

You may have a shorter fuse and get angry easier. I am getting angry thinking about people waking me up, and I don't even work nights anymore. If you offend someone because of your night shift temper, explain your situation and apologize. Let them know it isn't easy being a night shift zombie. Hopefully they can understand. If not, help them by calling them a dozen times throughout the night and keep them up. See how they feel the next day as a case study.

If you are already a nurse, then this chapter should have resonated with you. If you are a new nurse, now you know what to look forward to. It is important to understand what each shift is going through. I hear animosity between day shift nurses and night shift nurses. It is mostly due to a lack of understanding of how their nursing worlds function. We are all in this together, no matter what shift we work. Love on your day shifters and night shifters. We each have our hands full.

Understanding what to expect during days and nights is imperative to survival. Now that you know what to expect during your shift, let's talk about the most dangerous of male nurse ventures: "Hey, that nurse is pretty cute!"

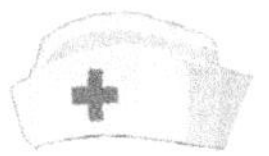

Dating

"The last time I trusted a nurse, she shot me in the ass
with Ativan and strapped me to a bed . . . Not too shabby."
— Unknown

WHEN YOU BECOME A MALE NURSE, YOU ENTER A WORLD full of dating potential. It's not quite *Grey's Anatomy* out there, but it is still pretty great. No matter your sexual preference, there will be opportunity for you as a nurse to find love, fornication, or whatever you seek. If you prefer women, then there will be a great opportunity since you are entering a world full of women. We are outnumbered, but this can be a very good thing.

Dating may be the most dangerous area of practice in nursing. Dating coworkers can bring about love, marriage, and happiness. It can also end in drama, anger, and destruction. You will learn things about women while working with them. They will tell you their dirtiest secrets at times. Women are vulgar, dirty, and sexual. If you don't believe me, just wait until you work with them. This is how you survive in the hospital dating pool.

You spend a lot of time with staff getting to know them. This happens even more during night shifts. There will be downtime where you get to know your coworkers. You already have something in common, as you are both in health care. Relationships can spring up quickly. On a hospital unit, information travels faster than in a high school. There is nothing nurses love more than gossip — especially relationship gossip.

Never, ever gossip. The less you say, the longer your relationships will last. The worst thing you can do is hook up with a coworker and tell everyone about it. You have to trust that if you tell anyone on the unit that they will keep a secret. A better rule of thumb is believing that if you tell someone, they will tell everyone.

I caution you to keep your business to yourself until it becomes serious. Some hospital units have policies against people in a relationship working together. This is another reason why it is better to keep the relationship on the down-low. If you like someone, then you obviously want to spend more time at work with them. You do not want to be forced to separate. You don't want to have to work opposite shifts or schedules. Be a relationship vault and you will have a lot more success in your dating life.

I worked with a young male nurse who was a little goofy, but a nice guy. The other nurses nicknamed him "Baby Huey," so that tells you he was considered the little brother type. He would say some awkward things at times, but everyone liked him. He was on a dating app and matched with the attractive house supervisor who worked nights. He asked her out to grab some food and she said "yes." Instead of Huey keeping this to himself, he decided the next day to tell all the female nurses on the unit about how excited he was to match and have a date with the hot house supervisor. She, of course, found out, and in less than twenty-four hours, the date was canceled — and Huey lost his chance to strike gold.

Keep the details to yourself. If the other person decides to share what you both are doing, then that is different. There is a good chance they will tell someone. Nurses are close and like to share what's going on in their lives. If it spreads around the unit, then it can be enticing to also share your experience. The safe bet is to just smile, shake off any questions, and keep the details to yourself. This will earn you trust with your partner and also keep you out of trouble. There is nothing worse than details spreading that your partner didn't want others to know.

Don't play with emotions. It is important to be honest from the start. If you are only looking to have fun, then make sure the other person knows that. If you are looking for more, then let them know. Honesty is the best policy here. Do not tell someone you are looking for a relationship and just be a player. You will ruin your reputation fast. Remember, emotions get the best of us, and even something that is supposed to be fun can turn dramatic quickly. If you are honest upfront, then you are in a better position to weather this dating storm.

If you play with emotions, lie, or cheat, it could be disastrous. Not only can you create an enemy, but also there is a good chance their friends and nursing posse will become your enemies. There is nothing worse than working with a group of women who want to see you burn. Like I stated in the first chapter, the lionesses run the unit. It's your goal to not get eaten. Don't mess with their cubs!

I met my wife at work. She was a travel nurse on the same unit I worked. We worked twelve-hour night shifts together many times, just the two of us. She was smart and sexy, and we really hit it off. She eventually invited me over for a massage; the rest is history. We were going on dates and spending time together for months without anyone knowing about it. When other staff would ask, I would either play dumb or laugh it off. I knew keeping my mouth shut and not gossiping would pay off. We got to work all our shifts together because no one knew we were dating. No one ever found out we were together until we left the unit and began traveling together. Keeping our relationship a secret was the best thing we did.

My best friend used to make out with the charge nurse in the linen closet at work. He used to tell me how awesome she was and how much fun they had together. That is the problem with nurses: they are really fun and know how to take care of people. We get sucked right in. Andy and Sara fell in love, and they now have four kids together.

I was working with my coworker Sarah when the new guy from the ED dropped off a patient and took a liking to her. Later that night, he sent chocolate through the tube station and a sweet note. It was so cheesy, and it was also an amazing move. She loved it! I didn't know what to think of Will at first. I even felt like a lioness. He was too smooth. It turns out he was a great guy, and they hit it off. Will and Sarah are now married, and Will and I also became great friends. An important side note is Sarah did not share her chocolate with me that night. I am still mad about it.

My Favorite Pick-Up Line for Nurses

**You are out and about and meet an attractive nurse.
Put on a big smile and say . . .**

**"Oh, I love nurses . . . they don't mind getting
in the dirty areas."**

If you do it correctly, then she will smile, nod, and say "yes."

Be careful — you might be married after using that line!

When I heard Huey matched with the house supervisor and had a date with her, I was astonished and excited for him. I then got the rest of the story on how he blew it by telling everyone. I felt a little ill because I have made this mistake before. If I could go back in time and warn poor Huey, maybe things would have been different. I could have given him advice. "Don't tell anyone about this. Thank your lucky stars and keep quiet!" I am hoping this book helps all the Baby Hueys out there. You all deserve a chance with the hot house supervisor. Don't blow it!

These lessons are tried and true. Dating nurses can be a fun and fulfilling experience, or it can be a disaster. I hope this chapter helps keep you out of trouble. In the next chapter, you will learn a male nurse survival technique that comes with a 100 percent guarantee . . .

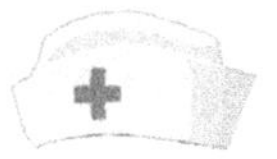

Warning . . . Don't Become a Nurse!

"I wear body fluids that aren't mine. I work weekends
and holidays.
I get screamed at and have my hands in other people's bits.
Tell me again how hard you work?" — Unknown

HOSPITALS SEEM TO ALWAYS BE SHORT-STAFFED, AND NURSES are leaving the profession. Why? Sure, nursing can be incredibly rewarding. You work and interact with some of the greatest people on the planet. You will meet some of the most passionate and caring individuals in the world. You get to take care of and contribute to your fellow human beings. You touch lives — and save lives. Why would anyone leave?

Now I get to burst your bubble. It's not always like that. It is different in the real world. Some of you probably heard sayings like, "Nurses are born to save lives!" or, "It must be so rewarding to be a nurse!" I'm here to tell you that nursing isn't full of rewarding experiences and grateful people. It is a tough job! It can break you down and beat you up. There is a lot about nursing that sucks! We have been undervalued and disrespected for far too long. This just might be the first book to tell you how it is.

This chapter is not intended to scare you away from nursing. (I hope you don't scare easily.) This is a long chapter because I wanted to get a lot of detail on these issues. My goal is to advise you on the hurdles you will face as a nurse. My other goal is to put them down here so we can work toward fixing them. It is about identifying the problems so we can make this profession better.

I often joke with the young patient care techs who are in school to become nurses. I like to mentor them on their nursing path. I offer my best advice to you now: don't be a nurse! Go and become a bartender at a fancy hotel or bar. Keep your eyes open. Find a rich man or woman to marry. Go and live a happy, rich life traveling the world! When I give this advice, I am only half-joking. I believe that could be a considerable life plan. If it is too late to find the right man or woman, there is always a chance to avoid this crazy profession. You have been warned!

I could fill an entire book with my frustrations about the nursing profession. I believe it is important to know what you are getting yourself into. I am giving you a 100 percent survival guarantee if you never become a nurse in the first place.

Disclaimer: The following examples are prevalent, but perhaps not everywhere. There are thousands of hospitals and units around the country. Some are good, and others are just plain terrible. What you will read here is very rampant in my experience as a nurse of over fifteen years. If you are a seasoned nurse, then this chapter should resonate with you. When you are a nurse long enough and work enough places, I promise you will see this and more. A lot of what you will read is responsible for the frustration and burnout of this profession. We cover how to survive burnout in the next chapter.

HOSPITALS

The first lesson to drive home is that hospitals are big business — every single one of them. They are in place to make money. I do not hate the idea of hospitals making money. How else would they pay us? I understand that a business needs money to effectively operate. This fact greatly affects our patient care and us nurses. Remembering that hospitals are big businesses will help you understand why and how hospitals function.

Nurses tend to forget that a hospital is a business. We want to believe that these institutions' only goal is to help people. We nurses are then treated like cogs in a wheel, and some can't understand why. Somehow nurses always end up bearing the brunt of hospital leadership's cost-cutting ideas. Many hospitals will aim to meet their bottom lines, skimp on resources, and use the least amount of staff possible. They use fancy words for "nurses getting screwed," like "benchmarking." Fancy words like these are created to compare all of a hospital system's units and staff ratios together. They look for creative ways to justify cutting back on staff and resources to save money. They don't care about nurses, the workload of a unit, or how it affects patients. How would they? Most people who run a hospital have never worked on a unit. Their highest priority is saving a buck. They do all these things and expect us to just smile and work harder. Most nurses just do it.

There are hospital systems that function under the guise of "nonprofit," but do not let that word deceive you. Every hospital is here to make money. A great example: The largest nonprofit hospital system in Utah started losing hundreds of millions of dollars during the beginning of the coronavirus pandemic.

In preparation for the pandemic, the hospital system chose to close down their surgeries and drop their hospital capacities in preparation for a sick wave that did not come. The wave did eventually come, but not until much later.

Do you know how they decided to make up for this lost revenue? Do you think the presidents, CEOs, and administrators went without pay? They didn't have to go in to work and risk their lives like nurses did. Hospital leadership decided to furlough nurses, ask for early retirements, and drop the 401k match of essential health care workers. They then adjusted the paid time off requirements so the staff received less paid time off. This disproportionately affected the more senior staff. The more senior you were, the less paid time off you now received.

They dropped the retirement benefit match of their essential workers in a pandemic and deducted their time off. They furloughed nursing staff and asked for early retirements from nurses. Then they cut staff down as short and tight as they could. The leadership of this hospital system made decisions that cost their *nonprofit* hospital system money during the pandemic. Essential staff and nurses were not at fault for that huge loss, but they paid the price. The nursing staff risked their lives and their families' lives coming to work during a pandemic. Their reward was losing benefits.

The pandemic eventually came to Utah in the fall of 2020. This hospital system had to bring in a large number of travel nurses to sustain the workload. They had to pay out loads of money for travel staff because they forced nurses to retire and nurses quit because of low hours and disrespect. They tripped over dollars to pick up dimes!

This is just one example in thousands of hospital systems' and nonprofit hospital systems' of lack of empathy for staff and patients. They study numbers and spreadsheets, not patients and staff. I have seen it over and over again in my career. To be in the nursing game, you have to know how the game is played.

ADMINISTRATORS

Hospitals are run by administrators. They are the leadership team creating policies, rules, and procedures for the staff to work under. There are amazing hospital administrators out there. Most of the great ones I met were nurses with lots of experience. The worst administrators were those who never worked on a hospital unit before and didn't understand what it meant to perform there. They seemed to care more about polls, metrics, and surveys than reality. The biggest frustration is administrators who have no clue how a unit or hospital really functions. Now, there are some administrators who have worked on a unit but moved up the ranks so quickly that they never got real experience. They don't know nursing, but they know how to say the right things and play politics. These administrators create rules and procedures that do not correlate with reality. My least favorite administrators are those who went to school for hospital administration or social work and never actually worked in a hospital or know what we do as nursing staff. It's like someone going to school for business but never running one. Theory is not reality. They only see from the outside looking in, and therefore they can't understand what we do.

Many of the policies and procedures these administrators enforce create additional work for the staff without creating any positive changes. From my experience, many administrators are reactionary. They don't make changes until an event takes place that then forces a change, despite staff members consistently pointing out the problem. An event happens and a decision is made to enforce a policy that makes everyone's job a little harder.

My favorite approach is for administrators to give out candy or cookies instead of fixing real problems like short-staffing or low pay. "Oh, you hate your job because we are incompetent? Here are some cookies. Happy Nurses Week!" They are out of touch with what is happening on the front lines of their hospital. It is endemic, and it is why so many nurses are leaving the field.

My wife, Jessica, was travel nursing at a facility in New Jersey that was an excellent example of administrators who ruin hospitals. Their staff was quitting, and they couldn't keep nurses. This was great for us because the pay for travel nurses was outstanding and they kept extending her contract longer and longer. They even told the staff to quit; they would just hire more travelers. This was proof that hospitals have the ability to pay nurses more money, but they just choose not to. As a traveler, we try and stay out of the drama, but it is hard not to get frustrated when dealing with incompetence.

Jessica would tell me that it wasn't a difficult place to work. The administrators created most of the problems for the staff. They ran their units short-staffed on purpose and allowed the cynical and lazy nurses to bully the new nurses. This is not a great way to give nurses a sense of pride for their hospital.

A favorite story she told me was what happened at their "Falls Friday" meeting. Every Friday, a group of administrators got together to talk about patient falls that happened that week. The staff that had a patient fall either had to show up in person or call in on the phone line. This may sound harmless, but it was a waste of time, energy, and brain cells. It was a justification of the administrators' jobs. They could look at the chart or talk to individual nurses if there was a problem with a fall. There were already protocols in place for reporting and charting. If anything was out of the ordinary, missing, or charted wrong, then they could track that nurse down.

They held this meeting at 9:00 a.m. every Friday, which was completely disrespectful to the night shift staff who ended their shifts at 7:30 a.m. This was a first sign to me that they were unaware, incompetent, or simply disrespectful to their staff. Working nights is difficult enough without having a meeting an hour and a half after the shift is over.

After a few months, they decided it would be mandatory to be in person on Falls Friday. It truly made no difference whether you called in or were there in person.

You just worked a twelve-hour night shift? Sorry, but you have to stay another two and a half hours to finish this meeting. Try not to fall asleep on the way home and kill someone. You have to work tonight? Looks like you aren't getting much sleep today. Oh, it's your day off? Get the kids to day care because you have a pointless meeting at 9:00 a.m. This is why people quit!

A great example of Falls Friday and administrators making things worse was an incident where a patient slipped and fell due to some liquid on the floor. An accident, but how do we prevent this? The administrators, with their wealth of experience, decided the solution was to ban patients from having anything to drink on the unit except for one in designated area. This meant no water in patients' rooms, hallways, or the common area; you may only have water in the kitchen. This is unheard of in other facilities and units. They didn't even know who spilled the liquid, and it was an isolated incident that had not happened before. All future patients must be punished for safety!

In fact, this solution was so absurd that Jessica actually was laughing when she told me this story because she thought they were joking when she heard about it. It wasn't until later when she was talking to a staff nurse on that floor that she found out it had actually been implemented. The nurses attempted to explain that this would actually increase patient falls, as psychiatric medications and dehydration do not mix, but it was implemented nonetheless. Guess what happened . . . they had more falls!

By the end of Jessica's travel contract, she had the second-most seniority on the unit. She was there for only six months, and she was second-longest employee — and training new travel nurses. The most senior nurse staff nurse was being pushed around a lot by management and felt disrespected and dispensable. By the time Jessica left this contract, the only staff member more senior than her was in process of looking for a new job. She was so over the place by the end of her contract that there was no amount of money they could pay her to stay.

There are many examples we have encountered in our careers. I could fill a whole book with just examples of bad management and administrators over my time as a nurse. Some of you will read this and relate to what I am saying. Maybe you have seen similar situations. Some of you probably have better stories than I do. If you work at a facility with great administrators, then this section can allow you to feel grateful for that. Bad administrators are the real pandemic in health care.

> **If you are an administrator reading this, then I'm sure you are a good one. I am sure you care deeply and want to do a great job. If this chapter causes you to pause or get irritated, then maybe it is a teaching moment for you.**
>
> **Take a moment to reflect; we all can be better. Perhaps you could shadow staff on each unit and position within your hospital to learn what it is like on the front lines in their shoes. Talk to your staff on the front lines and encourage them to be honest. Spend a day with housekeeping. Follow the nurses on a busy shift. Work a night shift and then go to a mandatory meeting at 9:00 a.m. It just might change the way you look at your job and your hospital.**
>
> **Poor leadership has been the number one cause of struggle and poor working conditions in every hospital I have ever worked in. We cover leadership later in the book.**

SHORT-STAFFING

Nurses are overworked. It is even worse when we are too often short-staffed. Staffing is an issue across the board. For my entire career, there has been a nursing shortage, and there is no one attempting to fix this problem. Nurses have a ton on their plates, and administration is constantly finding more jobs for nurses to do. If there is a new task or they must be a cut somewhere, it falls on the nurses' shoulders. Housekeeping doesn't want to take the linens off the bed to clean when a patient leaves? That's OK; the nurses can do it. We want to cut down on dietary workers? That's OK; nurses can deliver trays. We don't want to hire a phlebotomy team? That's OK; nurses can draw labs all day and night. I think it's become a normalized attitude in hospitals: "The nurse can do it." There is no end to the updates, policy changes, and tasks to keep up with. It is exhausting, and if something isn't getting done, then the nurses can do it. As a nurse, it feels like the only notifications we receive are what we are missing in our daily routine or what new task we need to add to our already one million other duties.

Nurses continue to take on more, and then we are often forced to work short-staffed. Nurses work with fewer nursing assistants or other nurses on the floor a lot. This means that nurses have to take on more patients and more duties than they should be, leading to increased stress and decreased performance. It is overwhelming, and it is a huge reason for frustration and burnout in our profession.

I firmly believe that nursing ratios should be revamped across the board. I have seen ratios improve since I started as a nurse. I know there are still places out there that stretch their nurses as much as they can. There are some positive implementations, like state law nursing ratios. I also understand there are circumstances out of a hospital's control, such as multiple call-offs for a shift. There are situations where you cannot control being short-staffed. For many hospitals and units, this is just everyday life.

The problem is when you are short-staffed, nurses are not happy. Nurses are not happy, so they quit, and then your remaining nurses are even worse off. It is a self-fulfilling prophecy. The sad part is not only do the nurses suffer, but so do the patients. There are times as a nurse we just have to pick up the slack. The problem is we are tired of picking up all the slack.

I have some ideas to improve staffing, and I believe this should be a bigger conversation in our profession moving forward. I think the coronavirus pandemic with nurses leaving the profession to travel or just leaving all together has exacerbated this already prevalent issue. Short-staffing is something everyone knows happens, but there is no long-term strategy to fix it. The governing bodies, universities and hospitals aren't working to get more nurses into the profession quicker from nursing schools. They continue to prolong degrees, mandate unnecessary bachelor's or master's degrees, and make it increasingly harder to get into nursing school. We need to change this so we get more nurses and develop them faster.

Hospitals continue to use Band-Aid tactics such as travel nurses and bonuses for nurses to pick up extra shifts without fixing the underlying problem. They assume it will fix itself. If you took that money and put more nurses on the floor, hired more assistant staff, and increased hourly pay, then you would keep and attract more nurses. I cannot imagine this is a revolutionary idea, but it somehow is missed in our profession.

Most of the units I worked on would improve drastically with one or two more nursing assistants to help out. Just one or two each shift — that's it. Hire more assistants and pay them more money. Overstaff on assistants. They work so freaking hard and make nurses' jobs so much easier. They deserve it. Do you know what it would be like if I wasn't pulled constantly for a pull up in bed, to clean a patient, or to run into a room to stop someone from falling when a bed alarm goes off? It would be a much different work environment.

I really believe in the team effort and having great ancillary teams to help us nurses. It makes a huge difference having a transport team, float pools, an IV team, a speech therapy team, a phlebotomy team, wound care nurses, etc. I think hospitals would do well to invest in and increase these divisions. There should be a goal to decrease a nurse's workload instead of increasing it.

My favorite idea would be a policy of staffing fairness. One thing you will learn as a nurse is that if your unit has a low census and not many patients, then you better send nurses home and cut down your staff. You better work within the defined ratios. We cannot work one minute overstaffed, or there is hell to pay. God forbid we have it too easy. It is the biggest taboo as a charge nurse to be overstaffed. Administrators will come and bring their wrath down on you. If we are understaffed, though, the attitude is that we should just suck it up, be team players, and work harder. At least we have a job, so we should be grateful for the extra work. It helps us grow as people. I hope you can read my sarcasm. Enough is enough!

I propose that if the nurses and techs have to work short-staffed, then they get to split the wages of that missing staff member. They would normally be paying for that nurse anyway, right? It would make me feel a lot better that if I am working my ass off, at least I am making more money. That unreliable nurse called off again and left us short? Now instead of wanting to slash her car tires next time I see her, I am excited because I got paid part of her wages for that shift. The shift sucked, but we split up that extra money. That sounds fair to me. Maybe just create a short-staffed bonus for your nursing team. I think this would help two-fold: the nursing staff would be happier, and it would force the administration to look at ways to stay well-staffed. If it hits their pocket books, then they pay attention. Maybe then we can eliminate the plague of short-staffing forever.

THE PAYCHECK

Money is not the most important factor when it comes to nursing, but it is very important. Like Zig Ziglar said, "Money isn't everything, but it ranks right up there with oxygen." Most nurses wouldn't place money as the number one or even number two reason on their hierarchy of professional needs. More important factors are things like company culture, good management, growth opportunities, workload, respect, and trust. When you don't fulfill on those needs, then the size of your paycheck greatly increases in importance. I believe that nurses and nursing assistants deserve a raise. I also believe that if you are in this profession, then there is nothing wrong with asking for more money. We work hard, and it is a tough job, so we should get paid well for it.

I learned a big lesson from being a travel nurse from 2020 to 2022: hospitals that were seemingly broke found ways to pay nurses large amounts of money to come and help. Some were absolutely huge sums of money. This proved to me that hospitals have the financial means and capability to pay nurses more money than they do now. There are hospitals adamantly fighting paying nurses more money, while their CEOs get multi-million dollar paychecks. It is ridiculous! Look at my example from earlier in this chapter where they cut down nurses and then brought in travel nurses. They could have just respected their staff and paid them more money. Perhaps the pandemic showcased the fact that we are really important and should be paid more for what we do.

WASTE

There is an incredible amount of waste in hospitals — wasted time, wasted resources, and wasted money. It took a few years to see these patterns, but when I began to realize the amount of waste in health care, it was discouraging. The biggest waste you will see is money.

The United States spends more on health care than any other country. We also have some of the lowest life expectancies, highest suicide rates, and most expensive technologies compared with all other developed nations.

The financial burden falls on the patients. The problem we don't see as nurses is the financial strain on the patient after they leave the hospital. There is so much waste on unnecessary procedures, tests, and interventions, and it hurts people.

Consider this example: I worked with a fantastic physician. She was a hospitalist, which meant she covered most of the hospital at night. She was very intelligent. Her downfall for me was that she would order every test, every procedure, and every intervention for every patient. She was too thorough. This sounds like a great thing, but it wasn't. She went over the top and ordered many unnecessary things. It seemed like every patient she admitted was put on telemetry to watch their heart. If the patient was twenty-two years old and had a broken arm, they got telemetry just to be sure.

One of her relieving hospitalists told us how much telemetry costs the patient — hundreds of dollars per day. He couldn't believe the cost. This proves that even doctors don't know all the costs of health care they prescribe to their patients.

This physician would take over and discontinue telemetry for most of the patients, many of whom didn't require it in the first place. He did this because it was not necessary and was costly to the patients. He was a great doctor. As nurses, we don't deal with the financial burden these patients have; that's another department. It is outside our radar. Most doctors either don't think about it or don't care. Some physicians I firmly believe add tests and interventions to make more money for themselves and the hospital. If you have ever been in the hospital, then you would understand the incredible costs it entails.

I have not been a patient at the hospital many times in my life. I vividly remember one occasion when I was sick and couldn't keep anything down all day. After a trip to the bathroom to vomit my ninth time and not being able to keep down water, I was ready for an intervention. I went to the ED at the hospital I worked at and received some IV fluids and Zofran. I was feeling better, as I assumed it was likely a short-term stomach illness. I had no respiratory symptoms, but they decided to do a flu test just to be sure. I was dumb enough to do it. A flu swab procedure means they take a long Q-tip and stick it up to your brain. I really hated it. To my enjoyment, I got the bill and found out that flu test cost $230. I hadn't reached my deductible yet, so that $230 was mine to pay. I can tell you it aggravates me just writing it here and now.

Another common waste in the hospital is keeping patients longer than necessary. "Let's keep them another day just to be sure." This happens so frequently, and it is a waste of time, resources, and money. I can't think of a single example where staying an unnecessary extra day was a benefit to the patient. It is even worse when the patient is a pain in the ass. Then it is a waste of our sanity as nurses. The physician decides to keep them another day because they often feel like it. I have seen this more times than I can count. The patient is fixed, stable, and ready to leave. The doctors decide to keep them just to be sure.

According to Health Catalyst, "Improving and reducing length of stay (LOS) improves financial, operational, and clinical outcomes by decreasing the costs of care for a patient. It can also improve outcomes by minimizing the risk of hospital-acquired conditions."[3] I really believe this information should be shared with all doctors and administrators across the country. It is not common practice in our health care system.

These are just a few examples of the millions of unnecessary costs being thrown down the line to our patients every day in hospitals.

Another form of waste you will encounter is trash. We waste so much plastic and paper; it is insane. Computers have helped a lot in the waste department, and I am grateful for that. There are still some paper charting facilities out there. Hopefully they will be getting computers soon. I was introduced to a company attempting to recycle for hospitals. I began researching and taking notice of all the plastic we encounter and throw away. According to the Healthcare Plastics Recycling Council, "Health care facilities in the United States generate *approximately 14,000 tons of waste per day*, most of which is being disposed of in landfills or by incineration. It is estimated that between 20

---

3 "Systematic, Data-Driven Approach Lowers Length of Stay and Improves Care Coordination," Health Catalyst, November 6, 2018, https://www.healthcatalyst.com/success_stories/reducing-length-of-stay-memorial-hospital-at-gulfport.

percent and 25 percent of that 14,000 tons can be attributed to plastic packaging and plastic products."[4]

That is a lot of plastic. The good news is there are more recycling solutions happening with hospital initiatives toward becoming greener. As nurses, we are the front line of reducing waste. We can be better at using opportunities to save and manage our resources.

PATIENT SATISFACTION SCORES

Would you like a hot towel or mint with your pain medications? Here come the Hospital Consumer Assessment of Healthcare Providers and Systems (HCAHPS) scores. In 2006, HCAHPS scores — also known as patient satisfaction scores — were created, and nursing changed. The scores comes from a 27-question survey created by the Centers for Medicare & Medicaid Services in partnership with the Agency for Healthcare Research and Quality. The survey was created so patients could give feedback on the hospitals and care they received. Hospital scores are also public, so people can compare scores and choose where they want to receive care. Some survey questions include communication with nurses, hospital cleanliness, overall rating of hospital, and pain management (which changed to "communication about pain" after the opioid crisis of 2018; a conclusion could be drawn that HCAHPS scores contributed to this crisis).

In 2012, HCAHPS scores were tied to hospital reimbursement from Medicare. This means that if a hospital's HCAHPS scores suck, they lose money. Hospitals hate losing money, so

---

4 "Solutions for Hospitals," Healthcare Plastics Recycling Council, accessed February 14, 2022, https://www.hprc.org/hospitals.

they had to adjust. There were good changes that came from the patient satisfaction scores, such as cleaner hospitals, better food, and a better patient experience. They also created a big problem: hospitals became more worried about a good customer experience instead of what's best for patient health. God forbid we tell the patient something they don't like. We don't want to get a lower score and lose money. We need to make these patients happy. Most of this work falls on the front-line workers. This means you, the nurse.

> **"The prominence that the government now places on patient satisfaction survey scores has led hospitals to come up with creative ways to improve patient satisfaction. Unfortunately, some of them have no positive health benefits. For example, some hospitals, influenced by the commercialization of patient satisfaction, are providing patients with designer gowns and valet parking, leaving critics to point out the diversion of resources away from proven measures for improving patient care quality. Another example . . . describes how nurses are being coached by consultants to verbally inform patients they are 'closing the door and turning out the lights to keep the hospital quiet at night.' The sole purpose of narrating this activity is to influence patients' survey responses.[5]**

What does this mean for nurses like us? It means we get the experience of feeling like glorified customer service agents who pass pills. Nursing became more about how satisfied the

5 "Patient Satisfaction Surveys," NEJM Catalyst, January 1, 2018, https://catalyst.nejm.org/doi/full/10.1056/CAT.18.0288.

"customer" is compared to how can we take the best care of them and get them healthier. It perpetuates the feeling that we should be more robots than health care practitioners. We receive more policies and regulations to perform at levels where we don't have to use our professional judgment. How do we keep the patient as happy as possible? This plays on our mental health and frustrates even the best nurses in this profession.

There was a large wave of gratitude for health care workers when COVID-19 hit in 2020. It really was the first time I felt any real gratitude or love for what we do in a long time. We still deal with this issue of patient satisfaction versus providing the best health care for our patients, though. You are the face and voice of the hospital, and we need to make sure that the customer, oh I mean the "patient," is satisfied.

CHARTING

The ever-increasing documentation as a nurse has spiraled out of control. It seems like nurses spend more time documenting interventions than it takes to perform them in the first place. This has been an ongoing problem perhaps since this profession started. It has been since I started. There is a constant barrage of new documents, protocols, and boxes to check. We must double-, triple-, and quadruple-document for agencies and administrators to be satisfied. Most of the time this has little to no effect on the patient's outcome. This goes back to wanting perfect nurse robots rather than actual thinking and high-performing nurses. Countless administrators are being overpaid to come up with pointless documents and extra tasks for nurses to do. They justify their jobs by creating more work for us. A full overhaul should be done to minimize and streamline every hospital's charting and documentation systems. Look where we double- and triple-document and cut it out. This would save so much needed time, money, resources, and energy.

What can we do as nurses? I always suggest charting by exception. I see nurses spend hours and hours documenting every single detail of their day. They pound this into your head as a new nurse to terrify you into wasting your days away charting. Learn to chart the important stuff and figure out when you can skip the double-charting. It will save you time and brain cells and give you more time for the important things like patient care.

I wish I now could give you all the answers. Of course every profession in the world has its problems. These things happen in other industries too. You have bad organizations, jerk bosses, dumb rules, and waste in almost all working sectors. My main goal of listing this here was not to scare you away from nursing, but to highlight the destructive factors plaguing our profession. These are the reasons why health care workers are leaving. The first step to recovery is saying we have a problem. Maybe it's up to the next generation reading this book to fix these issues. Maybe this chapter can help improve our profession.

Did this chapter make you question your career as a male nurse? You needed to know it isn't all sunshine and rainbows, but I hope you are brave enough to keep going. The world needs more great nurses. You now know the biggest pitfalls in our profession. Maybe you can be the one to fix it. I do believe we can improve all these areas only with the right leaders. Maybe you can help make real change out there.

You've learned a lot of about what frustrates nurses. What happens when we burn out?

Chapter 11

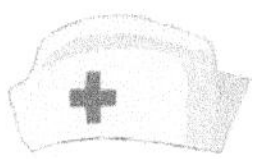

Feel the Burn . . . Out

"If we didn't have humor at work, what would we have? Ulcers.
We'd have ulcers." — Unknown

NURSE BURNOUT IS EMOTIONAL AND MENTAL EXHAUSTION that causes feelings of frustration, fuels a lack of motivation, and decreases a nurse's work efficiency. Burnout is becoming more and more prevalent. Some other names for burnout are "moral injury" or "compassion fatigue." I like the word "burnout" because it is the closest to how I feel in my emotions. I get fucking burned out! Whatever you call it, it is important to your long-term survival as a nurse to avoid or bounce back from burnout.

Burnout is a process, not an event. It happens when frustration builds and your patience diminishes over time. This happened to me on my little psychiatric unit, which I grew to love. I was a clinical supervisor, and life was good. I had the system down; my girl (now wife) would work every night with me, and she did all the hard work. You know I loved that. It wasn't a difficult place to be, and I enjoyed it. Then it began to slowly collapse.

It started like it does everywhere — from the top. A new CEO of the hospital was announced. He was a smooth-talking social worker who had no experience on a unit and didn't know how to run a hospital. This was an immediate red flag. He began implementing new protocols and procedures while ignoring the real problems — and causing new ones. It wasn't easy for him to see the big picture when he had no experience to lean on.

The second pillar to fall was our manager, whom I loved working for. She moved on to bigger and better things. It was great for her, but she left a big opening for who would take over.

A great manager can hold together a unit even in a bad system. Our unit director was told that she would now take on both jobs in the interim. She would be unit director and manager of the unit. This short-term Band-Aid turned into a long-term solution because the CEO liked the idea of skimping on the money. The problem with this was that our unit director was also a social worker. I have nothing against social workers, but she could not do anything to help us on the floor. She couldn't cover a shift, she didn't know what really happened on the unit, and she could not fix our nursing problems because she didn't understand them. This caused more and more frustrations among staff as time progressed. We began having staffing issues and increased safety issues.

My first course of action was to take my concerns to the other senior staff, who felt the same way I did. I then took my concerns to our unit director and other management. Our concerns fell on deaf ears. This caused me to begin feeling unappreciated quickly. I luckily worked with Jessica, so I was able to vent my frustrations, and we were able to talk about our worsening work environment together. It helped to talk with someone who understood.

Everything finally hit a point where we were fed up. I can't tell you exactly when that was, but it was close to when one of my favorite male nurses left. When he left, I knew the place was done for. Jessica and I decided that it was time to move on. There is only so much you can do, and it all fell on the poor leadership. We knew that the leadership was bad and wasn't going to get better any time soon. We decided to make a change and left for a travel nursing job. It was a great place to work, and so many simple little things could have saved it. The beauty of this profession is that there is so much opportunity for us. Once we walked out the door on our last day, it was all behind us. I'm not saying to just run when things get tough or there is conflict, but sometimes it is the only way to survive.

Nurses are often treated as expendable products of a hospital machine. When we do something about it and finally leave, the system acts shocked. They ask questions like, "Where is your loyalty?" "How can you do this to us?" I wish they would just treat us better and maybe this would hold some weight. At the end of the day, you have to do what is best for you, your health, and your family.

Burnout can show up any number of ways. If you feel yourself becoming increasingly frustrated, cynical, short-tempered, stressed just putting on your scrubs, or crying before, during, or after your shift, then it is time to take an evaluation. The most important part is recognizing the situation before you burst.

Burnout can occur for any number of reasons. You learned a number of those reasons in the previous chapter. Some more direct examples include extended exposure to short-staffing, poor unit management, conflicts with peers in the workplace, feeling bored, being stuck without a path for growth, or having to always clean up your coworkers' messes. It is usually not just one, but multiple stressors that cause burnout.

Being able to separate your work life from your home and family life is imperative to survival. If you are constantly thinking, living, and breathing your nursing career, it is easy to get overwhelmed and break. Nursing can be a high-stress, thankless job. If you are constantly living in that mindset, then you will burn out.

WHAT TO DO IF YOU ARE EXPERIENCING BURNOUT

1. Talk to someone you trust.

Express your feelings. Make sure they will not gossip and that they will keep it confidential. There is usually one wise and trustworthy nurse on the unit. If you don't have one of those, try a nurse who you know and trust somewhere else. Nurses are helpful listeners because they can relate. If you're in a relationship with someone not in health care, they may not understand what you are going through. This is OK. It can be frustrating when you want to vent to them and they don't understand. Don't take it out on them. If you want to talk about it, then go to someone who will understand. Sometimes a good venting session can be therapeutic.

2. Write out what is bothering you.

Getting it out of your brain and onto paper helps unload. You can throw it away or burn it after. This can also help you organize what is going on so you can solve it — that is, if solving it is possible. What we think of as a big deal loses its power when it is written down. Once you know what to fix, then go about fixing it. Men love fixing things. You can approach your manager or colleagues with solutions instead of being Mr. Cranky on the unit.

3. Work to fix the issues.

If it is a coworker, then you could try to talk to them in private about what is bothering you. Sometimes it is just a misunderstanding and can be worked out. If that does not accomplish anything, then talk to your boss and scheduler so you don't have to see them. If it is your boss causing you problems and you have spoken to them without resolution, then talk to their manager about it. Work through the channels to remove the cause of your burnout. You are tired and pissed off anyway. What do you have to lose?

4. Have activities outside your work that make you happy.

Find hobbies, family time, exercise, or games that make you happy and allow you to get your mind off work. This is very important because it allows you to decompress. It can give you the strength to deal with difficult situations when you return to your workplace.

5. Make a change.

The hospital, unit, or specialization may just not be right for you. It is not worth your mental and emotional health. Find another job, or move to another place in the hospital. It might sound scary, but the beauty of nursing is that there are so many opportunities and specializations for us. Don't ever let anyone make you feel bad if you are leaving for the right reasons. If you are burnt out, there is a good chance others are too. They aren't brave enough to do what you are doing. Prioritize your health over your job because it isn't worth it.

Burnout, moral injury, or compassion fatigue is lurking, waiting to pounce on you. I hope you don't have to experience it, but there is a good chance you eventually will. I loved the step-down ICU I started my career at, and I might still be there if they didn't close it and turn it into an orthopedic unit. There are great places to work out there, but you have to have the awareness to know if you are feeling burnout. Perhaps we can fix the big issues plaguing nursing to eliminate some of the burnout factors we all feel.

You have learned how to survive burnout, but what about the unspoken part of nursing we will never escape? How do you handle the awful patients who make you want to pull your hair out? How do you survive the wild ones?

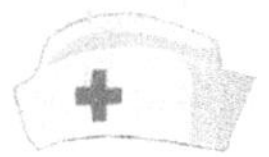

The Wild Ones

"You can't fix crazy. You can only document it." — Unknown

PEOPLE ARE NUTS! AND GUESS WHAT? WE ARE IN THE people business. Obviously, you and I are nuts because we are nurses. If you are saying, "I'm not nuts" . . . maybe you are the one exception, or you are probably lying to yourself. We all are. Sometimes we get to see miracles and people at their absolute best. Most of the time, we are dealing with people at their worst. This chapter is about dealing with difficult patients.

I consider difficult patients to fall into one of two groups. One is the people who need real mental health care. They have diagnosed disorders such as depression, bipolar disorder, schizophrenia, etc. Behavioral health nurses take care of these people as their specialty, but you will see these patients on medical floors as well. Many of the things you will learn here were taught to me through working on a behavioral health unit.

The second type of patient you will meet can be angry, difficult, abusive, annoying, med-seeking, violent, racist, manipulative, or just plain awful. Not everyone is going to be appreciative of your care. Some will actively fight against it. I wanted to cover this topic because no matter what you do in nursing, you will be dealing with difficult people.

I am a believer that the abuse we receive from patients needs to be addressed at a larger scale within the hospital's structure and policies. We should not be the punching bags, mentally and physically. This is also a cause of burnout: patients believe that since they are having a tough time, they can take it out on us. I believe it needs to stop. Nurses should be allowed to stand up for themselves. We are not quite there yet, but this chapter will help you maneuver these delicate situations. These difficult people show up everywhere in our profession, and you need to know how to work with them.

I picked up a lot of these tips and tricks from my wife, who is an awesome psych nurse. I met her when we worked on a small behavioral health unit together. I didn't know anything about psychiatric nursing, but she taught me a lot. It was interesting going back into medical-surgical nursing and using the techniques she taught me. These tips, tricks, and tactics are a combination of experience and her lessons to me. No matter where you work, they will benefit you.

THE MUSCLE

Men are generally sought when patients become more aggressive or violent. The female nurses will love having you around for these types of situations, especially if you are bigger. (This may be motivation for getting to the gym.) There are times when these individuals will calm down or de-escalate simply because there is a man talking to them. Use that to your advantage when you can. There also may be times when this does not work and ramps up their anger. They see a man, and they are looking for a fight. Know when to step back and allow them to calm down. Don't get hot-headed or try and dominate the situation because it isn't about you; it is about the patient. You want to be there for your ladies and back them up. Know how to keep yourself, your team, and your patients safe.

If you need to hold someone down or restrain someone, know how to do it properly. Many hospitals give training on how to do holds and restraints, as well as education on dealing with violent patients. I recommend taking this class no matter what department you work in. You never know when you will need it until it's too late. The other nurses will love working with you if they know you can keep them safe and deal with difficult situations.

DO NOT JUST TAKE OVER

Situations may vary, so you do not want to just barge in and take over. Our natural male instincts make us want to come and handle a situation. Tense situations arise, and we want to just jump in. Refrain from doing this. Strong women hate it when men jump in, thinking they can't handle a tense situation themselves. I have worked with many women who would kick my ass and yours. Men who think they should take over every situation will only make things harder. If you are working with a strong nurse, then follow your team lead and only step in when you are asked to do so. If they are floundering or you can see potential danger, then hop in. If you take any training in how to de-escalate a patient, you will learn that one speaker is all that is necessary. If you are not the primary nurse (or if they did not ask for you to step in), do not interrupt them. It will only make things worse.

PUT YOUR EGO AWAY

Do not get into power struggles with patients. It is not good for them, and it is unprofessional of you. In nursing, my philosophy has always been, "What will give me the least amount of headache?" This translates to, "What is the least amount of work I need to do to get my desired result?" This philosophy has never let me down.

For example, on a psychiatric unit, if a patient wants a snack and the rule is that they can't have snacks after a certain time, what do you do? If I know the patient — and know that if I say "no," it will result in an argument or worse — then I am probably going to give them a snack, within reason. I am not fighting with a psych patient at midnight over a graham cracker so he can wake up the whole unit. It usually will go something like this: "You know you can't have snacks at this time, but I'm going to bend the rule for you this once. You can have one snack, but that's it for the night." Sometimes I would say this with a smile, and sometimes I might be more serious. It depends on the patient. The patient is probably hungry because psych medications make you hungry.

On a medical unit, perhaps the patient has been here before and is well-known to the staff. They are here for pain medication and requesting it as early and frequently as possible. I can go in and fight this out with them, hold my biases against them, or try and break their habits. This would most likely lead to a poor relationship with the patient and increased work for me as the nurse. I instead put my ego away and work to create a plan to have a structured and productive shift where we both succeed in getting what we want. I will let the patient know the plan, medication regimen, and timing of the pain medications.

I will be firm with the plan, but empathetic. I will allow them to express themselves and listen. I will let them know when their next medication is due and make sure to be there at that time. This will lead to patient being happier with their care, and I don't feel manipulated or go overboard with the patient's medications. I will not let my ego or frustration get in the way of my care.

These examples can translate to all sorts of scenarios in our profession. The reason you put your ego away is because if you ramp this person up and they become angry or violent, it will be so much more work for you. You have to do phone calls to doctors, possible restraints, and lots and lots of charting. I have watched nurses pick fights for some of the most ridiculous reasons, and it only led to more work and headache on their part. That is the exact opposite of what I want to do during my shift. I want to calm things down and smooth it out so we all can make it through the shift with the least work and trauma possible. We get paid the same, so why not make the shift as easy as possible? This is why creative de-escalation tactics are important skills to have.

MANAGE YOUR REACTIONS

How do you control your emotions and give yourself time to react to an unruly patient? A powerful weapon in your arsenal is a being aware of your facial expressions and body language. Having control of these can work wonders. My wife taught me this from her psychiatric experience, where you cannot react to their nonsense. Work on controlling your body language and facial expressions so you are naturally nonreactive. If a patient is acting up or pushing your buttons, there is nothing better than to not react. It shows them that you will not give them the satisfaction of a reaction. It also allows you to collect your thoughts for a response. It may just give you enough distance to leave the room before laying a smack down on them and losing your job. All nurses with some years of experience have wanted to lay a smack down on a patient or two in their career.

My wife had a patient in the ED who was in a manic phase of bipolar disorder and also had borderline personality disorder. This patient wanted attention from any person on the floor. It was the middle of the night, and the patient was fighting sleep. The two nurses on were practicing the technique of benign neglect. The patient's needs were all attended, but there was no extra attention to be given. This patient attempted to get attention by putting herself against the glass of the nurse's station and melting down the glass while moaning. It took everything for the nurses to ignore her and not bust out into laughter. She then laid on the floor and called out their names. Annoying, but the nurses didn't budge. The last attempt was the patient laying a blanket on the ground and urinating on it (think of *The Exorcist*). She had never asked to use the bathroom and only did this to get a reaction. When she finally realized the nurses were not going to give her the satisfaction of a reaction, the patient went back to her room and finally went to bed. Sometimes the right thing to do can be messy!

You need to be aware of your limits and boundaries. Know when to step away when you may be at your wits' end. It is OK to pass this person over for a short break, or even for the rest of your shift. There will be certain patients who take us to the edge. Self-awareness is very important.

BE NICE!

This hails from one of my favorite '80s movies, *Road House*. One of my favorite scenes in the movie is when the main character, Dalton (Patrick Swayze), is first introduced to the bar staff at the Double Deuce. He gives them his three rules, his last being "Be nice!" He tells them, "I want you to remember that it's a job; it's nothing personal." This is the best advice for dealing with difficult patients. I recommend you watch the entire unedited scene.

Your job is to keep your patients safe and do your work. I frequently see nurses get upset, frustrated, or angry with awful people. I admit, they get to me. I remind myself of this scene, and it always helps bring me back. *"Be nice! I want you to remember that it's a job; it's nothing personal."*

DON'T GET BACK AT PEOPLE

"If what you're doing feels good, then you are probably doing it wrong." If it feels good, it is wrong! By this, I mean that if what you are doing feels like you're getting one up on a patient, or you're really "showing them," then it isn't the right move. It is interesting to think about: if it feels good to stick it to that person, then you aren't doing your job correctly. The goal isn't to get back at someone or "win;" that would be a power struggle, and no one wins power struggles. The goal is to take good care of your patient. Make the right choices, not necessarily the ones that feel good. You have to remember that these people are stuck in a hospital and you get to leave at the end of your shift. Look for empathy if you can find it.

LISTEN

People like being heard. They feel the need to express what has happened and to be understood, especially when they are feeling wronged. Many times I have come to de-escalate a situation and just asked the patient, "What's going on?" Give them a chance to explain. Active listening can help them regulate their emotions.

Active listening means that you pay full attention to what they are saying. Don't interrupt them and repeat back what you hear. Also, asking the right questions — "How should we handle this right now? What can we do to help you? What can we do to fix this?" — will give them a sense of control over the situation. That can mean a lot to someone when everything else feels out of their control.

I work with nurses all the time who will interrupt patients, give directions without listening, or get into a power struggles. This only worsens a situation and can escalate the anger and arguing. Remember, be nice.

KNOW WHEN TO STEP AWAY

Listening is important, but knowing when to step away is just as necessary. You do not have to stick around for two hours listening to a patient vent. Sometimes they feel like they have a right to all your time and attention. It is important to learn how to set boundaries and know when to step away. This is especially true when someone is pushing your buttons and you are ready to burst. Just step away. You can leave the room and the interaction. You can talk to your charge nurse or another team member and let them know you are unable to continue with that patient. It happens to the best of us.

KNOW WHEN TO ESCAPE

A great skill to learn is how to escape the room when the patient is attempting to keep you there forever. I believe most of the time they are lonely and want someone to talk to. You ask them about their medications, and they start telling you their whole life story. It feels rude to interrupt them, but now it's been forty-five minutes and you still have other patients to see. It is OK to interrupt them and say something like, "I really want to come back and hear the rest of your story, but I have to go see my other patients. I will be back soon, and we can finish up then. Is there anything else you need right now?" I watch countless new nurses get sidetracked and behind on their work because they do not know how to do this.

We often get a heads up if a patient is a talker and likes to keep the nurse in the room for long periods of time. A tactic we use is the buddy system. I tell my buddy nurse that if I am not out of the room in five minutes, then you come get me. They then can come interrupt us and say something like, "Hey Chris, can you come help me in my patient's room?" I then get to escape. The buddy system is a great resource when you need an escape plan.

SET EXPECTATIONS

Setting expectations is one of the best ways to kill problems before they arise. Clear, direct, and transparent expectations will alleviate so much stress in your career. Letting a patient who is very focused on pain medication know their exact medication regimen is a great practice. Let them know exactly what they will and will not be getting during their stay by being direct. It may upset them, but direct and transparent expectations will stop many problems before they start.

I have met my fair share of difficult patients. One young lady in particular stands out. In providing her care, I was able to incorporate many of the lessons you learned in this chapter. I was a travel nurse in a city outside of Los Angeles, California, and it was my turn to get the patient no one else wanted to take care of. You know it is going to be a fun day when multiple staff members ask you, "Have you had her before?" with that "poor guy" look on their faces. They then proceeded to give me advice on how to survive this patient.

This patient had been there for months off and on. She was as frequent a flyer as you could get. She was a young sickle cell patient who had a very particular way she liked to be treated. Sickle cell disease is a very painful and difficult disease to live with. I don't want this story to take anything away from that. It was this patient's coping mechanisms and abusive personality that was the problem. She was also a product of this hospital's policies and how they treated their sickle cell patients.

She was a long-term resident of this hospital. The administration and physicians created a monster. They created a system where many young sickle cell patients were given high doses of Dilaudid and Benadryl over long and consistent periods of time. They didn't test for sickle cell crisis at this hospital. They just trusted the patient's verbal pain status and gave high doses of addictive medications.

When the physicians decided it was time to downgrade these sickle cell patients to oral medications so they could return home, the patients would demand discharge and then circle right back through the same hospital's ED. They would be readmitted back onto the initial sickle cell protocol and receive large doses of IV Dilaudid. They would get to start all over again. It was insanity.

There were about five frequent flyers there. My patient wasn't the only one, but she was the queen. She was the most notable and longest-running patient. She had been there almost three hundred days in the past year — three hundred days in the hospital! A staff member told me it probably cost Medicare around a million dollars at this point, but I'm not sure how true that was. I assume he was probably close, with the amount of time she spent there. It was a testament to poor leadership, poor care standards, and poor boundaries.

I was in a different place in my nursing career at this point. I was old and crotchety and didn't really have any emotional stake in the game. I was there to do my job, not save the world, so my first thought was, "Whatever she wants, if it's ordered, let's do it." They already set the standard; I was just trying to have a good day. As I write this, I imagine she is there right now hitting the call bell early for her medication delivery.

She set an alarm on her phone to alert her when it was time for her IV Dilaudid. IV Dilaudid is the best medicine we have. It is ten times stronger than morphine, and she was getting a hefty dose every two hours. The doctors added a breakthrough dose if her pain extended higher. This meant she could have an extra dose of Dilaudid between her scheduled doses of Dilaudid.

She always needed breakthrough Dilaudid on schedule between her other doses. She had them written down and alarms set. You were in there every one to two hours throughout the shift. Even if she was sound asleep, that alarm woke her up long enough to call. She not only called early but also would call and call and call until her pain medications were delivered. Even when she knew it was too early, she still called. She was told by management and different hospital directors to respect the staff. It didn't change her behavior. She lived there and believed she was entitled to her customer service.

I understand that sickle cell pain is something I've never experienced and that I cannot relate to. I am sure she experienced sickle cell crisis during periods of these stays, and it was terrible for her. I know these medications helped her at certain times, but we couldn't distinguish when that actually happened. No one is in crisis every single day for months. These were all signs of addiction, manipulation, poor boundaries, and staff abuse.

The entire staff was tired of dealing with her at this point. They had caregiver fatigue. The first time I met her, I was taking her Dilaudid and Benadryl first thing in the morning. She proceeded to educate me on the proper way to give her IV medications. Normally, I would just say, "sounds good," and give the medications how it makes them comfortable. My immediate problem is how she instructed me that her IV medications would be given with a flush even though she had IV fluids infusing at a high rate. Normally, I wouldn't flush these medications unless I had to. The compatible IV fluids would flow the medication into her veins at a safe rate where I don't need a flush.

I gave the medication how I saw best. The first thing she exclaimed, shocked, was, "You have to flush it!" I told her, "No, it is flowing in with the fluids." She got angry and yelled at me that it is a doctor's order to flush her medication. I told her I had never seen such an order. She got even angrier, so I tried to calm the situation down. I said, "I apologize. Let me go look into it because I don't flush if there are IV fluids running."

If you don't know, the reason to flush Dilaudid or Benadryl in this situation is to make them go in quickly and produce a better high. Yes, Benadryl can give you a high if pushed quickly into the IV too. I talked to my charge nurse, and she told me that what the patient told me was, in fact, true. The doctors had made this a normal way of caring for her. They appeased and appeased this young woman to a place where she could have whatever she wanted. I don't have any ill will or dislike for this young woman. I actually blame the administration and physician team who refused to set boundaries and allowed her behavior and enabled her addiction. I hold them responsible.

If she became angry with her care, she would discharge and then go right into the ED and be readmitted. It was the wildest display of abuse on all levels. She abused the system, staff, resources, and patient care. The worst part is it all fell on the nurses and CNAs to deal with her on the front lines. We are always face to face with the poor decisions of the higher management.

My last experience with her before I left the assignment still blows my mind. She would periodically just leave the unit. She was reminded over and over again that this was not allowed because it was a patient safety issue. She would still sneak away. It finally came to a point where it became a hard and final rule. The manager stated that if she left the unit, then she was to be discharged. The patient was educated on the new standard, but she decided to leave the unit for over an hour unsupervised and without notifying anyone. We didn't know where she was, so our manager said, "OK, she is discharged."

When she returned, it became quite a scene. She was angry because she was being discharged and it was time to leave. She said she was going to leave but refused to take out her IV line in her arm. To me, this is a huge safety risk and infection risk. That IV needed to be removed before she left. I asked my manager, "What do we do? She won't let me take it out." I imagined security would come and help me do this before she left. My manager called the legal team to ask their advice. After this phone call, she said something that blew me away: "If she won't let us take it out, then she can leave with it. We can't force her." I said, "Wait, what do you mean we can't remove it?" She said, "I talked to legal, and she can go with it." I then watched this young woman with my self-diagnosed addiction walk out with a fully functioning IV line. California has some interesting regulations.

My next task was charting my butt off and making sure it was well-documented that none of this was my fault. My justification was that IV line was hospital property. We wouldn't let someone walk in and take a computer. We should have taken that IV, but the story has a happy ending. She returned to the ED and was promptly admitted to another unit in the hospital to be given her excellent customer service and high-end pain medication regimen.

I used every skill and tactic from this chapter. We learned earlier in this book that we control our attitude. I remembered what Patrick taught me: "Be nice!" She was going through a lot, and me getting irritated or spiteful would have only made it harder on everyone — especially me. I never tried to get back at her, and I tried my best to empathize with her. I gave her the care she wanted within the boundaries ordered by the doctors. It made our days smoother and everyone happier. I listened when she directed me to what she preferred and did my best to appease her within our agreed-upon boundaries. I was able to understand what was important to her and accomplish those things.

Lastly, I set whatever expectations I could. I let her know when I would be in with her medications and not sooner. I let her know what I would bring and when, and I allowed her to ask questions and also agree with those expectations. It achieved better days for both of us. She still abused the call bell, but not quite as much as normal. I do not think the hospital should have allowed her abusive behavior toward the staff, but that was not within my control. I do not miss her one bit, although I do hope she finds peace and health. This story is just one example of the willpower and strength we need to employ these skills and techniques when dealing with difficult people.

Learn and practice these simple skills. You won't have to look far to find difficult patients. They are often lurking close by or about to show up on your unit. If you are capable of handling yourself, then it will make your work life — and everyone else's lives — much better. You will deal with difficult people often. That's nursing. They will test your patience, your willpower, and your desire to give great care.

You have come a long way in this book, and I am proud of you. Now that you are becoming an expert male nurse, you can start telling everyone how awesome you are. Stop! It's a trap!

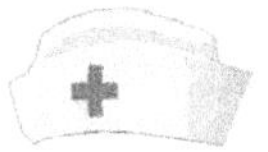

Chapter 13

Don't Get Too Cocky

"Hard work never killed anybody, but why take a chance?"
— *Edgar Bergen*

I LEARNED NOT TO GET TOO COCKY EARLY IN MY NURSING career. Even though it was a long time ago, I still remember this particular patient early in my career who would hit the call bell continuously throughout the day and night. It seemed like one thousand times during the shift, and it was ridiculous. He would call, and we would answer the call light and tell him we were on our way to his room. He would hit the bell again a few seconds later, before I could even get into the room. It was incredibly frustrating. This sort of thing will drive you nuts. Truth is, I wanted to shove the call bell where the sun didn't shine. I still get nightmares about call bells. The dinging can haunt your dreams. This particular gentleman was a full test of my patience. I was able to keep my cool that night, and we both survived.

They had been rotating him with different nurses because he was so mentally exhausting. There will be times when it takes everything in you to be calm and nice. You need to know your limits.

I came back in that night excited to have the night off from him. In my mind I already had my turn with this guy. Lo and behold, it was my lucky night. I asked, "Why do I have call bell guy again?" The charge nurse said in an attempted sweet tone, "Well, it is because you can handle him and this other nurse can't."

It was the first time I felt punished for being a good nurse. It was also an educational moment. I ran my butt off with this guy all night while the other nurse had a nice, smooth shift. She sat on her ass while I ran my ass off. We made the same amount of money. I have no problem running and working hard, but that isn't the point. I have a hard time taking the lion's share of work just because I can handle it. I believe in taking my fair share of bad patients. We all get our turn, but you don't want to be the go-to guy in every shitty situation.

This wouldn't be the last time this happened to me. Difficult patients and undesirable assignments would come back to me because I could handle them. I found that early in my career I would get the annoying or disruptive patients. I would ask why I get so lucky to have the difficult people. They would say, "It's because you can handle it." There are those nurses who freak out and have a hard time under stress. Why they became nurses, I have no idea. Why should I be punished for it? Sure, I could handle these situations better than some nurses I worked with. I have a great temperament for these people. The problem is that I don't want to be working that hard all the time. I do not want to be the one dealing with the crappy assignments. So I learned a thing or two that I am going to teach you here.

Getting punished for being a good nurse happens. Sometimes you can't help it. If you like doing the hard work all the time, then don't take my advice. You should want to be a great nurse. I'm just suggesting do it on the down-low.

Be good, but don't broadcast it everywhere. Don't be a cocky nurse. It is OK to have fun with it, but don't get on the radar. Women love bringing cocky men down a peg or two. If you come on the unit like the king of nursing, it might put a target on your back. You should be humble. We talked about the jungle: don't give the lionesses a reason to bite.

You don't want that extra attention because you may find a nurse who wants to prove to you and everyone else that you aren't that great. They are lurking and waiting. Do not give them the opportunity.

If you are the guy always solving problems, showing off your skills and claiming how great you are, then you will be the go-to guy. The problem is you then receive extra jobs, a heavier workload, or the worst patients.

This may seem contradictory to other things I have taught you in this book. You would think you want everyone to know that you are the best. It isn't true. You want to make sure your nurses know that you are good and have their backs, but you don't want them to think that you are so amazing that they work you to death. It is a little bit of an art form, but it's worth understanding. If you are humble with your skills, then you will have a more enjoyable nursing experience. It is important to be a skilled, loved, and, most of all, humble nurse.

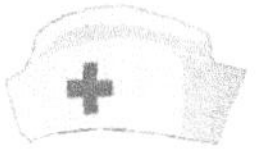

Chapter 14

Want to Travel?

"I haven't been everywhere, but it's on my list."
— Susan Sontag

TRAVEL NURSING IS A HOT TOPIC. IT IS ONE OF THE BEST ways to see the country while you work. You can make a lot of money doing it. Travel nursing is a great opportunity if you know how to do it correctly and have the temperament for the trade. As a travel nurse with multiple assignments under my belt, it is important to give any aspiring travelers the survival techniques I have learned over the years. I know of many great travel nurse experiences, but also some real horror stories. If travel nursing doesn't interest you, you can still learn a thing or two from this chapter. Most nurses have an idea about travel nursing, but don't really know what it entails or how to do it successfully. This is your guide.

THE GOOD

You get paid more — sometimes way more. The money is the best part about travel nursing. This has especially been true the past few years. The money has been awesome! Most travel assignments are around thirteen weeks, with some shorter at four or eight weeks. I learned that you can survive anything for three months or less. The time really does go by fast. If you do a good job, a lot of times you can extend your contract for longer contracts. You have the control because if you don't like it there, you can just leave when your contract is over. You don't have to deal with the politics and drama on the unit because you are only there for a short time. If it is a bad place to work or has nasty people, you get to make your money and leave. It's awesome! You get to go home, and those people have to stay.

You will get to meet new people and experience new things. Most of the time, the unit and employees are just excited that you are there to take care of people. Every hospital has annoying policies and tedious (sometimes just stupid) rules that don't matter. As a traveler, it is easier to ignore the insignificant ones.

In March of 2020, I was working as a part-time nurse while the coronavirus pandemic was ramping up. The country had shut down, and they needed nurses. My wife and I took travel nurse contracts across the country in New Jersey not far from New York City, which was exploding with COVID-19 cases. It was a hot spot. I took an emergency contract that started ASAP, so I could only give four days' notice that I was leaving. I had to pack up the car and head across the country to New Jersey from Utah almost immediately.

I asked my manager to move me to a PRN or "as needed" position so I could take the job. I was only working part-time anyway, and I moved from PRN to part-time shortly before this all happened. I told him if he didn't need me as PRN, I would kindly resign. The money was way too good to pass up. I sent him a professional and respectful email. I said that I understood it was short notice and that I was sorry to leave him this way. He instead fired me because he was angry. I don't know how he fired me because I said I resigned.

The new job paid three times what I was making at the place I just left. It was a huge pay increase, which is why leaving didn't bother me much. The hospital had plenty of staff, and I was willing to put myself at risk for the reward. I was a travel nurse for the next eight months. I made more money than I would have in three years at the hospital. The hospital I left was just fine, and it was one of the best career decisions I ever made.

THE BAD

You will be thrown into the fire. A lot of these hospitals need travelers because they cannot keep staff. Most of the time, this means it isn't a great place to work, or people would not be leaving. Sometimes they just need extra nurses to implement new charting systems or to open a new unit.

You will not have a full orientation, and you have to be a quick learner. You may be needed to float between units. If you are a nurse who needs a solid routine, then this will be difficult. It is not as easy as being a regular staff nurse, but the perks outweigh the downsides if you can handle them.

It was now April 6, 2020, and I made it to New Jersey from Utah. My wife and I had just got into town one day earlier after driving over two thousand miles, so I was tired. My wife's hospital was letting her orient the whole week online because of COVID-19. I was jealous. I was told to show up a half-hour early. Some places I have worked in the past gave me one or two days of orientation, and others gave me a week. It really depends on the hospital, and you don't know until you are there.

I arrived at the address I was told to show up at. The place was dark downstairs, as it wasn't a hospital, but a long-term acute care (LTAC) facility. I didn't have an ID badge to get in yet, so I thought, "Well, maybe I am supposed to be at the main hospital to orient."

I drove five minutes down the road and paid to park in the garage. I found a group of travelers in the lobby and a lady with a clipboard. She was very nice and told me, "You aren't on my list, but come with us. We are doing an infection control presentation, and we will figure out where you go." I followed along because it isn't unusual for a hospital to be unorganized.

I went through this presentation on how to sanitize and take off my gowns and gloves. After, everyone was going to a computer training class. The educator told me that I wasn't on her list and to go back and check where I should be. She told me to call if I needed that class or they had me coming back. I was thinking in my head, "Well, this is great!" but I have traveled before and this is not that uncommon. Sometimes you have to roll with the punches and, hey, I was getting paid anyway. I got back in my car and drove back to the original building.

This time it was 8:00 a.m. and the lights were on in the lobby. I walked in and let them know I was a travel nurse and was pretty sure I was supposed to be there. The lady running the front desk called the nurse supervisor down. She was a pleasant but tough middle-aged woman with a harsh voice from smoking a few packs of cigarettes per day. She had a straightforward demeanor and a no-bullshit attitude. I knew we would get along.

She was in charge of the LTAC facility that day and had no idea who I was. I figured it was a normal thing for her to be out of the loop, as it looked like they were doing the best they could under the circumstances. I was still not sure if I was in the right place, and she was not sure either. She stated, "We will find something for you to do." I assumed we were on our way to meet someone who knew what was going on. Since it was my first day, I expected to follow someone around and help out. I would learn the charting system, workflow, and protocols. The usual first day travel stuff; nothing too exciting. Boy, was I wrong!

We walked onto the floor at about 8:30 a.m. If you know what a day shift is like, then you know this is a busy time. The floor was buzzing with medications to be passed, patients to be assessed, and vital signs to be taken. They were also dealing with a new COVID-19 protocol every day. Everyone was running around when I got there. I had never worked at an LTAC facility before, but I had worked years in hospitals, so I thought, "How bad could this be? It's all good. Just a little different, but I'll survive." I was wondering which of these people in all this madness I would be following that day.

The supervisor took me over and said, "Here's your medication cart. There is your hallway," in a most matter-of-fact tone. The look on my face probably said it all, but in a sort of state of shock, I said, "Uh, OK." She then walked away. I got the message that I was here and it was time for duty — no orientation, no unit overview, no idea what I was doing.

The overwhelmed nurse I was taking over for came over and handed me the medication book. She didn't do anything down my hallway yet, or explain anything. Yes, this place had a medication cart with all the medications in it. You pushed this cart around the hallway and pulled the medications out of medication cards with a week's worth of pills in it. The narcotics were not in a sophisticated computer, but in a box in my cart. We opened this box with a key that one nurse was responsible for. The charting was paper, and the medication record was a book of patients and a grid to put my initials on. It took me fifteen minutes to understand what the medications were and when I was to give them. Good thing I didn't take that computer class at the hospital because that would have been useless. I was back to the Stone Age. After fifteen minutes trying to decipher the medications in the book and when to give them, I spent the next ten minutes looking over the medications in my cart. The last thing I wanted was to give the wrong medications on my first day.

I had a moment I will never forget, and it's great advice for any nurse. We talked about not panicking, and I took my own advice. I closed my eyes, took a breath, and said to myself, "You are making a lot of money. Keep them alive, and keep them off the floor" (meaning don't let them fall).

I took my medication cart to the first patient's room and worked through her medication list. These were elderly people with a lot of medications. I worked my way around the hallway and learned through asking a lot of questions, rolling with the punches, and using my experience to guide me. I survived!

The second day on the job, I was standing at my cart pulling medications and trying to be less overwhelmed than the day before. I saw one of my patients being run down the hall in their bed and onto the elevator to be taken to the COVID-19 floor. Apparently all the COVID-19 tests were coming back from the lab, and most of these patients were positive for COVID-19. The funny thing was that no one was telling me they were taking my patients away or where they were going. They were just going by me to the elevator. I was like, "Wow, there goes another one of my patients." Did I tell you that you had to go with the flow as a traveler?

WHAT DOES IT TAKE?

To be a travel nurse, you will need around one year of experience. Some travel companies will take less, but be careful: you must be comfortable being thrown into the fire. When I say "fire," what I mean is getting onto a unit with very little training where you don't know where most things are, which doctors to call, the proper protocols, or the normal workflow. You must get into the flow quickly without losing your mind. I believe that this takes experience. You want to know how to successfully complete shifts without drowning before you go traveling. To be a good travel nurse, you must be able to work without becoming overwhelmed. You need to know how to prioritize time well and focus on what is important during your shift.

CHOOSING A COMPANY

Once you have some experience and are ready to travel, you need to find a good company. Travel companies hire recruiters to set up the contract between you and the hospitals. All hospitals go through a third party, so you need to find a good company and a good recruiter. There are a lot to choose from, and not all companies are the same. Some pay less than others but have better services. Some pay better but have a limited supply of work.

Be careful looking at company sites. If you put your information in, here come the calls. The floodgates open, and your number is out there on the internet. If possible, I would ask other travel nurses what they recommend and their experiences with their companies. Make sure you talk to nurses you trust and get a few opinions. Make sure to use them as references when you apply because they usually get a bonus for recommending their company to you. But remember, just because they are a travel nurse doesn't mean their recruiter or company are any good.

You will learn what questions to ask so you can do your own research. Travel companies and recruiters make money off of you, so you are definitely the asset here. You want to make sure to get the best experience you can. It can feel overwhelming out there, so this is a list of what I look for in a company.

Things to Look For in a Travel Nursing Company

- **Health benefits start on day one**
- **Great pay equal or better than competition**
- **Professional staff**
- **Honesty in what they offer**
- **Assignments in the places you want to travel**
- **Good reputation**
- **Will pay for state license, if needed**
- **Travel stipends (covered travel costs to drive or fly to assignments)**
- **Good reviews**

CHOOSING A RECRUITER

Your recruiter is your lifeline to the company. They want you to be happy because you are their moneymaker. If you have a recruiter who does not understand this, get a new recruiter. They work for you, but this doesn't give you the ability to abuse them. You will be working hard and making them money on assignments, so make sure they work hard for you too.

> ### Things to Look For in a Recruiter
>
> - **Professional demeanor**
> - **Good communication**
> - **Honest and does what they say they are going to do**
> - **Promptly answers calls, texts, or emails**
> - **Cares about you and doing a good job for you**
> - **Responds well to questions or problems**
> - **Has your back if a hospital or company does not fulfill their promises**
> - **Well-organized**
> - **Willing and able to go after a particular job you want quickly and effectively**

CONTRACTS

You've got a great company and recruiter and found a location you want to travel to. The pay looks great, so you say, "Hey, put me in for that hospital, please." The recruiter submits your profile to the hospital, and they check out your resume. You may do an interview, or they may just see how awesome you are and say "yes!"

Your recruiter will send you a contract. You are able to ask for whatever you want in terms of days off, shift preferences, and more. If you need time off or anything important, then make sure it is in your contract. Do not take anyone's word for it — not your recruiter's word or the hospital's word. If it is OK with them, then get it in the contract. There are so many times they try to switch times, switch shifts, or deny time off after you start. If you need it, then get it in the contract. You don't need every detail there if it is something small, but if it is important, make sure it is in there. When you sign the contract, it's time to travel.

ON ASSIGNMENT

Your company and recruiter will make sure to get you the information for where to show up and what to do. They deal with any credentials you need before you arrive. It can be a scramble for blood work or drug tests, but they set it up and cover the costs.

Your first day is usually a hospital orientation of some kind. These orientations can be one day or a week. You usually get enough time to be able to learn the work, but not much more.

There is a good chance you will be liked immediately just for being a guy. It is a great thing. Use the skills I taught you in this book and you will thrive on the assignment. Many times, if they like you and still need your nursing abilities, then they will offer a contract extension. The new contract is separate from the original, so you can negotiate new pay rates, time off, shifts, and more. I have been places where travelers had been working for over two years in the same hospital through extensions.

Even the bad is still pretty great when it comes to travel nursing. I worked eight weeks at that place in New Jersey with a whole team of travelers. We worked the COVID-19 floor together and became very close. They were some of the best nurses I have ever worked with. We were in the trenches together, and I will never forget our time there. We took excellent care of our patients, many of whom were there with us for weeks or months. We were the only people they saw some days. There were days it was just two nurses running a hallway of twenty patients. We had to be a team or we wouldn't make it — no nursing assistants, just us. I wiped more butts there than I had in my prior five years as a nurse. It was the hardest I have ever worked and the most money I've ever made. That is what it is all about — going all in. You have to be willing to work hard and take the punches as a traveler because that's why we get paid the big bucks.

I was curious if I could go back to work at the hospital I was fired from when I took the travel contract. Eight months later, a travel nursing contract opened up at the same exact hospital system I was supposedly fired from. COVID-19 was just ramping up, and they needed nurses. This was great news for me. I succeeded in getting the contract and was back at the same hospital system making over double the money as a traveler than I made as a staff nurse. It did not matter that my old boss fired me or if he was mad. I did what I thought was right for me and my family, and it was the best decision I ever made. There were other nurses who told me, "I wish I could do that."

Travel nursing is a great way to see the country and make great money doing it. We are in a high-demand profession, and you can take advantage of that through travel nursing. It is my hope that if you choose to travel, this chapter helps you have a great experience. Now, what is the one thing we all desperately need in this profession?

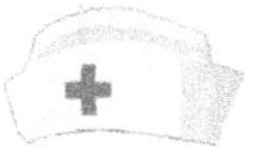

Chapter 15

Will the Leader Please Stand Up?

"The key to being a good manager is keeping the people who hate me away from those who are still undecided." — Casey Stengel

THE NURSING PROFESSION IS STARVING FOR GREAT LEADERS. The level of leadership in an organization is the main cause for the success or failures we endure as nurses. We talked a lot about administration and the frustration they present in this book already. Leadership is the number one skill we need to improve to make a big impact on the nursing profession. As men, we have an advantage to move into leadership roles rather quickly if we choose to.

If you have a high-functioning nursing unit with happy staff, then they have a great leadership team. If you have a poorly run unit with miserable staff and people leaving, then you will find the cause is always terrible leadership. In my experience, when staff decided to quit, it was almost always related to management or morale issues rather than a higher salary.

I have experienced many bad units all over the country and many different specialties. It always falls on the leadership. If

you become a better leader, then your career will improve —
and so will the nursing profession as a whole.

As a travel nurse, I am the guy they pay the big bucks to
when a unit can't keep staff from leaving. I get to see things
from a different perspective. It doesn't take long to identify
why people are unhappy. It usually falls on a handful of easy-
to-fix problems that management cannot see or chooses not to
fix. The main solution is always better leadership. If the unit
manager is a strong leader, then it doesn't matter if the hospital system is crap; it will still function strong. I have seen many
well-run units in bad hospital systems. Why? Leadership! The
opposite is also true. You can have an amazing hospital system,
and if the unit has a bad manager, the unit will flounder.

Every nurse should be interested in leadership. Whether
you are brand new or have been a nurse for a long time, it is
valuable for you to learn leadership. Most nurses aren't taught
how to be leaders. The good news is you can be a leader any-
where in this profession. These skills and knowledge will help
you be a better nurse and a better teammate.

I worked for a small orthopedic unit for over a year that
was running great. We had a strong manager and a happy and
competent team of nurses and nursing assistants. This unit was
so smooth that it ran itself. Then, it was time for the unit manager to move on to bigger things. I joked that the new manager
could come in the morning, take a nap, do meetings, ask how
the day is going, and head home. It was the easiest manager
position I ever saw. We had the unit rocking!

Instead of the administration making a smart decision and
choosing an internal nurse who currently worked on our unit
or in the same hospital, they chose an outside candidate. He did

not have a lot of experience, but he was a good friend of someone in administration, which is why he got the job.

He immediately started rubbing everyone the wrong way. He broke every rule of leadership you will learn here. Upon meeting everyone on the unit, he told us he was here to really improve things. Wait, he never worked a shift on our floor and was here to fix everything? You remember from Chapter 1 how much women hate this. He never even shadowed a shift on the floor. He proceeded to change scheduling requirements, procedures, holiday work requirements, and our staffing metrics. It appeared that anything we used to do was about to change.

Rather quickly, we began having more holes as people quit. As a manager, he would be expected to help out and fill those holes. He told the staff that administration advised him he is not allowed to do patient care. Nursing managers are the last line of backup. Managers jump in and work when the staff is too short. They are there to run this unit no matter what. We caught this manager in his lie because when we brought this to administration, they said he absolutely can do patient care. His lies began to stack up.

He immediately lost our respect and trust. Once you lost trust and respect, it is over. He also showed us that he wasn't willing to do the work. Leaders lead from the front. Senior staff began taking concerns to him and attempted to guide him. We were there to help. He either shut us down or talked about us behind our backs. When confronted with issues, he deflected or assigned blame to others. He checked every box of what it takes to be an awful leader. The good news is that the lionesses run the jungle, and this was not going to go on for long. This manager lasted less than six weeks on the unit. This was a smooth-running, efficient nursing unit. He broke every rule of leadership in the book. Maybe this chapter will help the next generation of managers and leaders to not make the same mistakes.

First, great leaders don't have to always be liked, but they absolutely need to be respected. When you climb the ranks of management, being respected as a leader is more important than being liked. Leaders know they need to get their job done and that not everyone will be happy about it all the time. Do you want your peers and team to respect you? To earn respect, you have to give respect. What is respect? Respect is listening and being empathetic to others. Letting others come to you with problems and concerns without getting defensive. Making sure you allow them to speak and not interrupt them. They will feel respected, and this will lead to a good working relationship.

Respect is trusting your team to do the right things. Trust is instrumental in gaining respect. If you can't trust your team to get their jobs done, then that's on you as a leader to train them or replace them. You have to trust your people and believe in them to be successful. They need to know they can trust you too. They need to know that when something happens, you will be there to back them up.

Respect is also not talking behind people's back. This is a common occurrence in nursing. Don't fall into the trap of talking behind your team's back. Be a professional. Professionals take problems directly to the source.

What happens if you lose that respect? The best path is to admit your mistakes, apologize, and ask your team to help you be better. Humbling yourself and asking forgiveness is so rare that it can help reset and begin building back lost respect.

Great leaders don't ask their team to do anything they wouldn't do. Are you willing to get your hands dirty? If you want to be respected, then your team needs to know you empathize with them and are willing to do the hard work too. When you refuse to help or divert responsibilities that are your own, then you lose your ability to lead. Be willing to jump in and help your team. Empathize with them when they are frustrated or implementing a new policy. Get in there and teach them how it is done. You don't have to do their jobs for them, but it is important for them to know you would if necessary. Do you jump in and help? Does your team know you are there for them? Do you have their backs when a problem arises?

I have a friend who was an Army nurse. She worked her way up the ranks at a prestigious university hospital and is the essence of a great administrator and leader. I have always heard great things about her, but her real-life front-line work blew me away. When the coronavirus pandemic started, she was the director of the Emergency Department. When those patients started rolling in, do you think she was doing video calls hiding at home like many other administrators I experienced? No! When COVID-19 hit, she was in the ED every day with her staff. She came in early so she could update the day shift coming on and the night shift leaving. She kept them informed on procedures, policy changes, and safety plans. She was right there on the front lines with her team. She showed her staff that they were all in this together and that she was there for them. Do you think they worked hard for her? You know it! That is a true leader, and we need more like her in the nursing world.

People want to know they are being heard and cared about. If a manager does not listen to their team or care about them, then they will lose them. I believe leadership is all about listening. If you are observant and ask the right questions, you will find the answers you need. Make your team understand that it is safe to bring concerns and questions to you. Let them know that it will not be held against them. Work to fix these problems, or be honest about why you cannot. The staff will love you if you can take criticism and work on improvements. Do you shut down concerns? Do you listen to your coworkers and team? Do you look at ways to improve the communication on your unit?

Honesty and integrity are integral parts of leadership. It is a pretty easy concept: do what you say you are going to do when you say you are going to do it. If you lie to your nursing team and lose that trust, then you lose your ability to lead. Let them know what you expect from them and hold them to that standard.

Does your team trust you? You must have your staff's backs. They have to know you are there for them. If they are going to try their best and something happens, are you there for them? They need to know that you will give them the benefit of the doubt and trust their judgments. It is your job to help them improve and learn from mistakes. When there is backstabbing or playing favorites, it spells disaster. They will never trust you, and you will lose your leadership abilities. Are you honest with your team? Do you have integrity at work? Can they have an open dialogue with you and know they won't be punished for it?

Being a great leader means taking responsibility. A huge problem in this profession is the lack of accountability in leadership positions. Administrators and managers tend to look down for problems instead of looking at themselves and how they can improve. When mistakes happen, a leader looks at themselves first. If your team is failing, it is because the leader failed them. A great leader will have their team wanting to improve and do great work. Of course there will be individuals who make mistakes. How does your unit or hospital function as a whole? Is it running smooth? You can take credit for that. Are staff constantly leaving and unhappy at work? You can take credit for that too. When a problem arises, do you blame others or yourself first? Take full responsibility and be a great leader.

I had a nurse manager I loved. She always told me the truth, whether it was good or bad. She was willing to jump in and help, listened, and took responsibility for any problems. I loved working for her.

Here's an example of her leadership. I was not completing a form that was required to be documented every night. It was the third place I charted the same information, just like the other two places before it. It was triple-charting. I had put off documenting it for a few weeks because it was just an unnecessary form. One day she came to me and said, "Hey, I know this form is stupid, and it is double- or triple-charting. You guys already do this, but can you please fill out this form for me? I know it is extra, but if you don't, I get in trouble." My response was, "Of course I will fill out the form." I happily filled out that stupid form every shift. I didn't do it because it was important, or because I cared one bit about the hospital's protocols. She empathized with me and then explained to me why it was important. She already had my trust and respect.

I filled that form out for my manager because she was straight with me, and I loved that about her. That is a real leader. I want to know you understand where I am coming from and how I feel. After that, I will do anything for you.

Nursing is starving for real leaders. The right leadership is the way we improve our profession and create great working environments. Develop your leadership skills and help others become great leaders. We face many problems in this profession, many of which have been outlined in this book. If you commit to being a great leader, then you will be doing your part to improve nursing for all of us. You know how to be a leader, but how do you stay in the nursing game for a long time?

Chapter 16

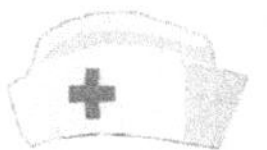

Take Care of Yourself

"Self-care is giving the world the best of you, instead of what's left of you." — Katie Reed

THE ONLY WAY TO ENSURE LONG-TERM SURVIVAL IN this profession is to take care of yourself. Our mental, emotional, and physical health is imperative to long-term success. I remember the first time I started meeting nurses who worked in the hospital for twenty and thirty years. They were overweight, angry, and could barely walk with their back problems. They were hardened, badass nurses who were busted up by the nursing lifestyle. I thought, "Wow, maybe I don't want to be a nurse for a long time." I realized it's not just nursing that beats them down; it's not taking care of themselves that does it. It is a hard work environment. You would think that being in the "health" field, you would want to stay healthy. This is rarely the case.

You will be around sick people with every disease and ailment you can think of. You want to make sure that your body and immune system are in tip-top shape. This is more important than ever in today's health care climate.

We are all very busy people. You must make taking care of yourself a priority not just on days you work, but every day.

There are physical, mental, and emotional aspects of health that we need to focus on daily. They all work together, so doing good things for your physical body will help you feel better mentally and emotionally as well.

HOW DO YOU TAKE CARE OF YOURSELF PHYSICALLY?

1. **Exercise.** There may be nothing harder than going to the gym and exercising before, after, or around your nursing shifts and on your days off. Some days you are on your feet all day, running and gunning. We all know why exercise is important. You must make it a priority.

2. **Eat healthier.** This may be one of the most difficult things to do on a unit. There is junk food around all the time. There always seems to be donuts, cookies, or pizza ready to be eaten. As men, we are often great garbage disposals for junk food. This is especially true when you work night shifts. There are times where all you crave and consume is junk food. It is OK to have the junk as long as it is in moderation. Work on eating healthier so you can take care of yourself — and others — longer.

3. **Practice proper body mechanics.** Don't hurt yourself. This seems self-explanatory, but nurses get injured all the time. Back injuries are one of the most common injuries for nurses. It might seem easy to try and save time doing things yourself, but an injury is not worth it. Make sure to ask for help — and use that help. Back problems suck and can be a lifelong injury. Make sure to stretch as well. Keeping yourself loose and limber helps with overall health and

helps avoid injuries. Did you know that some hospitals will not help with medical bills if you do not use their proper protocols and sustain an injury? Proper body mechanics are essential.

4. **Sleep.** This can be a difficult task as a nurse. Working long hours, especially if you work night shifts, can really mess up your sleep schedule. Try your best to achieve seven to eight hours of restful sleep each night. Get blackout curtains, earplugs, or a good eye mask if you need them. These can be worth their weight in gold.

5. **Take your vitamins.** Keep your body and immune system in top shape. We need it now more than ever. My personal favorites for immune health are vitamin D, B complex vitamins, vitamin C, and zinc.

6. **Drink water.** Hydration is very important. It is easy to forget to drink water when you are busy. Most people live their lives dehydrated. We do not drink enough water. They say to drink half your body weight in ounces — if you are 160 pounds, that would be eighty ounces of water per day, or ten eight-ounce glasses. My favorite way to drink water during my shift is to chug a cup every time I walk by the fountain or water fill station. Many units have a dietary room where we fill water pitchers. Each time I go there, I make sure to drink a glass of water real quick. I recommend limiting the soda and drinking more water. There is always time for water and bathroom breaks if you manage your time properly.

HOW DO YOU TAKE CARE OF YOURSELF MENTALLY AND EMOTIONALLY?

1. **Breathe.** Sometimes you need to stop and take a deep breath. I can't tell you how many times this has helped me anchor myself back to reality. When shit was hitting the fan, this was my saving grace. Take a deep breath.

2. **Practice gratitude.** When it is hard, tiring, and frustrating, gratitude is a great tool. Being grateful for your job, why you are here, or the people around you can help change any situation. This is not only helpful at work, but in every aspect of your life. Find your reasons to be grateful.

3. **Have hobbies.** You have to have activities outside of work that you enjoy doing. It is important to be able to decompress. Have reasons *why* you work hard.

4. **Meditate.** This is an amazing tool to help clear your mind and balance you. Mental health is so important, and nursing is a taxing profession. It is easy to find meditations online, and there are many applications available. Sometimes just five minutes with yourself can really help.

5. **Prioritize relationships.** Seek out good relationships and work hard to keep them. You want to make this a priority in your personal life as well as in your work relationships. Work will be more enjoyable if you have people you enjoy being around.

6. **Take vacations.** My advice is always to take that vacation. The hospital and unit will be there when you get back. It is important to step away and refuel. Sometimes a vacation is all you need to find happiness and purpose at your job again.

7. **Learn to laugh.** You must have a sense of humor in this line of work. It may surprise you what you are able to joke about after a few years as a nurse. Most nurses I know have a messed-up sense of humor. It is a way to decompress in a stressful environment. It is important to be able to laugh, joke around, and enjoy yourself in the chaos. It might just keep you sane.

My first travel nursing assignment was on a state prison floor. It was my first time in a new hospital, and it tested my mental and emotional fortitude. I had no idea what I was walking into.

It was intimidating the first time I went through a double-door system and I showed my ID to the guard. I was on the locked unit, and it was my job to take care of a floor of dangerous inmates. There were a number of guards on the floor, and you had to always take one into a room with you. This became extremely annoying when it was busy because you would have to wait for a guard to become available. The guards spoke very direct, and at times it felt like I was being talked down to. I realized later it wasn't on them; it was just the culture.

The patients were shackled by their ankles. Everything you took into the room, you had to take out because they would make weapons out of anything they could. An interesting note I learned is that they would put these items up their butts — a practice called "keistering" — and take them back to prison with them. It is crazy what you can fit in your ass and make into a weapon.

It really sucked if you forgot to grab something while entering a room. You had to pick up all your stuff, go get what you needed, and carry it all back in. Most of the inmates were pleasant because the nurses were there to help them. They also got a break from prison.

There was a particular inmate I took care of who was the most awful human being I have ever met. They never tell you what the inmates were in jail for because they didn't want you to have negative feelings when you cared for them. I heard he had done something pretty awful though, which only added to my dislike. I'm not going to sugarcoat it: this guy was a disgusting asshole. He was stabbed in the stomach in prison and refused the nasogastric tube. This led to him perforating his bowel and needing total parenteral nutrition (TPN) to survive. This is nutrition through your IV every day — thousands of dollars per bag that California taxpayers were paying for, every day. This guy had been there for seven months when I met him. I started counting up that cost.

Now, I don't believe money should be put in place of someone's life. I just tell you this because thoughts like these were creeping up later, and they might creep up on you at some point.

I knew mentally and emotionally I wasn't in a good place. He was miserable and abusive to everyone who took care of him. This guy wanted his IV Dilaudid pain medication every four hours on the dot. If you were five seconds late, he was calling, and he was pissed. Hell, he was pissed all the time, no matter what. None of the regular nurses wanted to deal with him anymore, so I was given him almost every day I worked.

I had only been a nurse three years in a big teaching hospital. I had never dealt with anything like this before. I was younger and less experienced than I am now. Thinking back, I could handle it much better now. I wish I had had this book to help me. He could smell the timidness all over me and preyed on it. This guy wore on me. I always gave him great care and was verbally abused for it.

I'll never forget my last day of my travel assignment. I should have been ecstatic, but instead I was miserable. I was sitting there in the afternoon stewing because this patient was on my last nerve. I was thinking about how awful he was, how much money he was costing the world, and other unpleasant things. It was wearing on me, and I was bitter. I was mentally and emotionally burned out.

Then all of a sudden the charge nurse said, "Hey Chris, you are being sent home early. Give report." I jumped out of my chair, and everything changed. I knew as a traveler, I still got my full day of pay even though was being sent home early. I skipped out of there knowing I would never see that unit or that awful guy again. It is amazing how fast you can change your state. I went from miserable and bitter to happy and excited in an instant. It proved to me that my attitude really was under my control. I was actually the one in control.

I wish I could go back and give myself the advice, "Fuck that guy. Don't take it personally; it's just a job, and he is not worth your stress." I wish I knew some of these mental and emotional exercises to calm myself down and get in a better state. Things like breathing, showing gratitude, and learning to laugh. It would have allowed me to be more confident in myself. Maybe I could have even had fun with it, or gave him some attitude back. He may have even liked me for it. I mean, he was miserable, and I wasn't going to change that. It is easy to emotionally and mentally break down. I learned how to take care of myself in all these areas, and it has led to being a better nurse and having a more enjoyable career.

Mental, emotional, and physical health is as important as any aspect in long-term survival as a nurse. These lessons translate not only to your job but also to your home and family life. Improving one of these areas can have a ripple effect on your life. If you want to be a finely tuned nursing machine, then you have to keep that machine in tip-top shape. You need to be ready for anything, move quickly, and not get overwhelmed to have a successful, long-term career. This is how we do it. Take care of yourself out there.

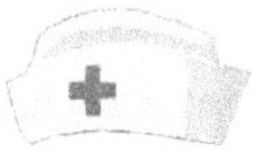

Chapter 17

Be a Great Nurse!

"Life doesn't require that we be the best, only that
we try our best." — H. Jackson Brown Jr.

THE WORLD NEEDS MORE GREAT NURSES. THIS PROFESSION is far from perfect. I believe that we can improve nursing from within with great nurses who really care. The world needs us — and it needs us to be great.

We don't just want to be nurses; we want something that fulfills us. We want to be excited to go to work and help people. We want to make a difference. Most of us got into this profession to contribute. Life is more meaningful when we are fulfilled.

It doesn't take much to be a great nurse — only a few seconds. It only takes a few seconds to be a bad nurse too. Bad nurses aren't bad people. Bad nurses just don't care about the little details and the extra seconds. It is the attention to details that make the big difference.

Do the little things right. Clean up after yourself. Get your work done so the next shift doesn't have to pick up after you. Do your tasks. Take care of your patients. Care about your team and take the steps to back them up. Take the extra second to do the right things. Choose to thrive instead of survive. Do the best you can for the time you are there.

There will be times you leave a shift feeling overwhelmed. You feel like you missed something, and it eats at you. You go home and have nightmares about it. It happens to the best nurses. There will be times you worry and wonder if you completed everything you were supposed to. Twelve hours can fly by in the snap of a finger. There is so much going on that it can be hard to keep track. It can be hard to get it all done.

The most important thing is knowing that you did your best. Nursing happens twenty-four hours a day, seven days a week. It doesn't all rely on you. Did you work hard? Did you help your team when they needed you? Did you take the extra seconds to do the right things? Did you get the important things done? If the answer is yes to these questions, then you were a great nurse and you can sleep well after your shifts. You can rest your head knowing you did your best.

If you apply what you've learned in this book, you are well on your way. I hope this inspires you to be the very best nurse you can be. You are a hero! Being great is a choice, so choose to be great.

Conclusion

"It is a skill to work this hard and
make it look this easy!"
— *Chris Lengle*

"HIS PENIS IS FALLING OFF!" . . . WHEN I WAS 19 YEARS OLD, I was halfway through nursing school and dreaming of being done. On one clinical day, we were in the hospital on a medical-surgical unit. I was paired with an annoying student who talked a lot and acted like she knew everything. We had one patient we were assigned to care for together. The gentleman we had was a sad case. I don't remember the name of his disease, but he had something like calcium depositing in his capillaries blocking off his blood flow. His whole back was a giant bedsore from shoulders to buttocks. It wasn't because of neglect, but because any pressure caused a wound. He was blind, and his fingers and toes were black and necrotic like they had frostbite. He was pretty much in a coma. It wouldn't be long until he passed away.

We were bathing him and the annoying student said, "Oh my God. His penis is hard like a rock. Touch it." His penis was also necrotic. His penis was dead and eventually was going to fall off. I can't imagine anything worse as a man. I declined and said, "No, that's OK. I can see it. I'm good." I was thinking, "Why the hell would I want to touch it?"

At the end of the day, we were doing our review with the nursing instructor and other students before we left. As we were reviewing our day, the annoying student said, "Yeah, Chris wouldn't touch the necrotic penis." I gave her my best "What the fuck?" glare from across the room. My teacher said, "You didn't touch it. Come on with me."

She marched me in the room and made me touch this poor dying man's necrotic penis. Walking out, she said, "I did that because you will never see something like that again." My response was, "Yeah, thanks," trying to hold back my sarcasm and "What the fuck was the point of doing that!" tone. Yes, this really happened, and yes, I wore a glove!

During that time, I was still living at home and sharing a bedroom with my twin brother. I was nineteen years old and wasn't ready to grow up yet. (Really though, do guys ever really grow up?) My brother was a snowboard bum while I went to nursing school. There were many times I thought, "Why didn't I just become a snowboard bum too? Why am I doing this?"

A few nights after this exciting day at the hospital, my brother awoke to me talking in my sleep. He heard me mumble and then yell out,

"His penis is falling off!"

The next morning, my brother — with a weird and concerned look on his face — asked, "Bro, what the hell were you dreaming about last night?"

I said, "What are you talking about?"

He said, "You were talking in your sleep and yelled, 'His penis is falling off!'"

As he stared at me concerned, I searched for the answer in my brain. It took me a minute to realize what would have caused this crazy dream. Apparently, the necrotic penis traumatized me more than I realized at the time. I explained to my brother what happened at the hospital and having to touch the dead penis. We had a really good laugh about it, and he couldn't wait to tell our friends about my nightmares.

As a male nurse, you will see, hear, and experience things you will never forget. You will see the best and worst of people, be burned out and frustrated, and find best friends along the way. You will learn a lot about yourself and others. You will learn to laugh at some really messed-up things. It all comes with the territory.

This book truly was a labor of love. I hope you got enjoyment out of it as well as practical and important lessons for your nursing career. By finishing this book, you now have the tools to defend yourself and survive. Revisit this book or a specific chapter when needed on your journey. Go make us male nurses proud.

***

I would love to hear your personal survival stories and experiences.

Please send them to
chris@danconia.gold.

Acknowledgments

FIRST AND FOREMOST, I HAVE TO THANK MY AMAZING WIFE, Jessica. You were not only my early editor, but you also motivate me every day to be great. You somehow could make sense of me mixing the past, present, and future in my storytelling and fix my mistakes. You just know how my brain works, and I couldn't have done it without you.

My mom and dad, who led me into nursing and were always there for me. I knew I could do anything because you were there to support me.

The rest of my family — Suzie, John, Ruby, Chuck, Lori, Penny, Robin, Garrett, Bryan, Mandy, and Zippy. I love you all!

Woodrow, my little Westie dog. You were my writing partner, and sometimes you wanted belly rubs or to play with your toys while I was in the zone. It was OK, because you are so damn cute! We made it work, great job bud!

My editor, Anna Bentley. I got very lucky finding someone who was so good at her job and so honest. I still can't believe you charged me less than your original quote. I am so glad I found you and would recommend you to anyone.

My cover artist, TK Palad, who did a phenomenal job with my cover. You made my vision look even better than I could have imagined. So glad I found you on Fiverr!

My book interior designer, Sue Balcer. I not only loved you were from Pittsburgh, but also that you did a fantastic job with the interior of my book.

Corie Shultheis at UPMC Shadyside School of Nursing. Thank you for getting my graduation photo from 2006 for this book. You were so kind, and I really appreciate your help. Without you, no one would have been able to see my baby face.

Stacy Dymalski and The Memoir Midwife. I am so grateful you were teaching with the Park City Learning Center and I was able to attend your class. Your book and wisdom helped me to avoid the pitfalls and self-publish this book. I don't know if I could have done it the right way without you.

Kyle Montag, thank you for the marketing advice and letting me bounce ideas off you. I really appreciate your friendship!

My boys on the front lines, who are some of the best damn nurses I know — Andy Austin, David Huber, Walter Gillis, and Will Samsky. Thank you for your input and insight on this book as it came together. It is amazing to have your friendship for all these years.

Kevin Sosa and David Adcock, my all-time rock stars. You are the most badass nurses and the only guys who read my book front to back when I sent it out. None of my other guys finished it, but you guys did, so beers are on me! Love you guys!

To the young male nurse who inspired me to write this book: thank you for your dumb comments and making this whole thing possible.

Lastly, to all my female nurses who took care of me, kept me out of trouble, and taught me the ropes: you are the real heroes and why I was able to write this book. I wish I could list off all of your names, but this would be too long of an acknowledgment page. If we worked together, then you know who you are. Thank you. You are amazing!

Bibliography

Borrelli, Lizette. "Random Acts of Kindness Raise Dopamine Levels and Boost Your Mood." Medical Daily. April 26, 2016. https://www.medicaldaily.com/random-acts-kindness-sweet-emotion-helping-others-dopamine-levels-383563.

Health Catalyst. "Systematic, Data-Driven Approach Lowers Length of Stay and Improves Care Coordination." November 6, 2018. https://www.healthcatalyst.com/success_stories/reducing-length-of-stay-memorial-hospital-at-gulfport.

Healthcare Plastics Recycling Council. "Solutions for Hospitals." Accessed February 14, 2022. https://www.hprc.org/hospitals.

NEJM Catalyst. "Patient Satisfaction Surveys." January 1, 2018. https://catalyst.nejm.org/doi/full/10.1056/CAT.18.0288.

Smiley, Richard A., Clark Ruttinger, Carrie M. Oliveira, Laura R. Hudson, Richard Allgeyer, Kyrani A. Reneau, Josephine H. Silvestre, Maryann Alexander. "The 2020 National Nursing Workforce Survey." *Journal of Nursing Regulation* 12, no. 1, Supplement (April 1, 2021): S1-S96.